Trauma-Informed Yoga for Pain Management

of related interest

Yoga and Science in Pain Care
Treating the Person in Pain
Edited by Neil Pearson, Shelly Prosko and Marlysa Sullivan
Foreword by Timothy McCall
ISBN 978 1 84819 397 0
eISBN 978 0 85701 354 5

Pain Science—Yoga—Life
Bridging Neuroscience and Yoga for Pain Care
Marnie Hartman and Niamh Moloney
ISBN 978 1 91208 558 3
eISBN 978 1 91208 562 0

Yoga Therapy as a Creative Response to Pain
Matthew J. Taylor
Foreword by John Kepner
ISBN 978 1 84819 356 7
eISBN 978 0 85701 315 6

Applied Yoga™ for Musculoskeletal Pain
Integrating Yoga, Physical Therapy, Strength, and Spirituality
Jory Serota, C-IAYT, LMT, NKT
ISBN 978 1 83997 882 1
eISBN 978 1 83997 883 8

TRAUMA-INFORMED YOGA FOR PAIN MANAGEMENT

A Practical Manual for Simple Stretching, Gentle Strengthening, and Mindful Breathing

The GreenTREE Yoga® Approach: Building Safety, Supporting Empowerment, and Maintaining Simplicity

Yael Calhoun, MA, MS, E-RYT
with **Mona Bingham**, PhD, RN

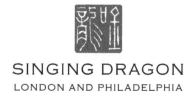

SINGING DRAGON
LONDON AND PHILADELPHIA

First published in Great Britain in 2024 by Singing Dragon,
an imprint of Jessica Kingsley Publishers
Part of John Murray Press

2

Copyright © Yael Calhoun 2024

Illustrations copyright © Sam Tresco. Many thanks to Sam Tresco, White Gorge Designs. www.whitegorgedesigns

The right of Yael Calhoun to be identified as the Author of the Work has been asserted by her in accordance with the Copyright, Designs and Patents Act 1988.

Front cover image source: Shutterstock®.

All rights reserved. No part of this publication may be reproduced, stored in a retrieval system, or transmitted, in any form or by any means without the prior written permission of the publisher, nor be otherwise circulated in any form of binding or cover other than that in which it is published and without a similar condition being imposed on the subsequent purchaser.

Disclaimer: The information contained in this book is not intended to replace the services of trained medical professionals or to be a substitute for medical advice. The complementary therapy described in this book may not be suitable for everyone to follow. You are advised to consult a doctor before embarking on any complementary therapy programme and on any matters relating to your health, and in particular on any matters that may require diagnosis or medical attention.

A CIP catalogue record for this title is available from the
British Library and the Library of Congress

ISBN 978 1 83997 800 5
eISBN 978 1 83997 801 2

Printed and bound by CPI Group (UK) Ltd, Croydon, CR0 4YY

Jessica Kingsley Publishers' policy is to use papers that are natural, renewable and recyclable products and made from wood grown in sustainable forests. The logging and manufacturing processes are expected to conform to the environmental regulations of the country of origin.

Singing Dragon
Carmelite House
50 Victoria Embankment
London EC4Y 0DZ

www.singingdragon.com

John Murray Press
Part of Hodder & Stoughton Limited
An Hachette UK Company

The authorised representative in the EEA is Hachette Ireland, 8 Castlecourt Centre, Dublin 15, D15 XTP3, Ireland (email: info@hbgi.ie)

*To Aram of Cedar Brook. And to everyone interested
in exploring new ways of managing pain. ~ YC*

*To all those who serve in the Armed Forces, may you
find these tools and suggestions useful. ~ MB*

Acknowledgments

Many people helped this book come to be. The GreenTREE Yoga® Board has provided support for our program development for over 15 years, for which I am grateful. A special acknowledgment to Gina Jensen, LCSW, who shepherded the trauma-informed yoga program at Salt Lake City Veterans' Affairs, and whose untimely passing left us striving to nurture all the seeds she had planted. Jamie Clinton-Lont, NP, Medical Director at Salt Lake City Veterans' Affairs Women's Clinic, asked me to develop a program for pain management. Many veterans came to my classes and taught me as I fine-tuned the program that grew to six classes a week. Mona Bingham, PhD, RN, a retired Army Nurse Corps Officer, attended my classes for years, and provides the medical anchor for this book. Yvette Melby, LCSW, E-RYT, and I collaborated to create the pain management program for refugees, translated into six languages. A special thanks to all the wonderful people in my workshops, classes, and trainings who have provided the feedback that inspired this book.

Many thanks to Margaret Clayton, PhD, APRN, FAAN, Professor Emerita, College of Nursing, University of Utah, for her tireless manuscript reviews. Others who shared their time, talents, and expertise include Elizabeth Q. Finlinson, LCSW (trauma therapist and our yoga model), Louis Allen, MD, FAAP, Cameron E. Hatch, LCSW (trauma therapist), and Katelyn D. O'Farrell, PhD (exercise physiologist and yoga teacher). A group of dedicated yoga teachers, working with populations with pain concerns and/or in trauma recovery, spent many hours reading the text, practicing the sequences, and sharing their thoughts. So to Rebecca Carroll, RYT 500, Mariann Bourland, and Emma Powell—many, many thanks. As I always say: teamwork. Finally, a heartfelt thank you to Sam Tresco (www.whitegorgedesigns.com), for insisting he understood the concepts before doing his clear and inviting artwork.

Contents

Preface 9

Introduction 11

Part I: The Science of Healing

1. The Basics 19
   Why Science Basics Can Inform Your Program 19
   What Is a Neuron? 20
   What Is Neuroplasticity? 22
   Types of Pain 25

2. Movement 30
   Moving: Why It Matters to Pain Management 30
   Moving: How We Do It 32
   Moving: Doing It Better 37

3. The Mind–Body Connection 42
   The Mind and the Brain 42
   Gate Theory 44
   How We Process Pain: Perception and Emotions 45
   Stress and the HPA Axis 47
   The Breath 50
   Polyvagal Theory 55
   To Learn and to Unlearn 57
   How Yoga Puts It All Together: Mind, Body, and Breath 59

Part II: Making It Trauma-Informed

4. What Is a Trauma-Informed Approach and Why Is It Important? . . 67

   Language 69

   The Room 75

   Classroom Management 78

   All About You: Teacher, Clinician, or Healthcare Provider 79

   Assists 82

   Teach to Empower 83

   Ways for You to Practice Your Trauma-Informed Teaching 88

PART III: Simple Practices for Everyone

5. Introducing the Sequences 93

   An Overview of Part III 94

   Trauma-Informed Language 95

   Seven Teaching Points 96

   A Closer Look: Practice Sequence Descriptions 99

   In Case You Missed It... 101

6. One- to Five-Minute Breaks 105

   Introduction 105

   Breathwork (photos on p.262) 107

   Simple Stretching 111

7. Thirty-Minute Practices 115

   Outlines and Practice Sequences 115

8. Sixty- to Ninety-Minute Practices 189

   Outlines and Practice Sequences 189

Part IV: Appendices

   Practice Sequence Photographs 239

   Resources 263

   Author Bios 265

   Endnotes 266

Preface

This book is the result of my being tasked with developing a pain management program at Salt Lake City Veterans' Affairs, where I had started a trauma-informed yoga program for veterans seven years earlier. I had seen how the trauma-informed yoga had helped with pain management, even though the referrals to my classes were based on clinical diagnoses of post-traumatic stress disorder (PTSD) and military sexual trauma. To develop a specific program for pain management seemed both an exciting challenge and a strong need.

How I developed my program explains how I came to write this book. The veterans in my classes had both physical and emotional pain, so I knew that I needed a mind–body approach. My task was to develop a program for pain management and not for specific pain issues. I started reading everything I could about yoga and pain. I found books on the topic, but none struck me as the answer for my program. It was not until I had a clearer vision for the class that I was able to identify what was lacking. Some books seemed geared toward those with established yoga practices doing more advanced poses and challenging sequences. The veterans with whom I worked would have been overwhelmed and discouraged. Some books lacked a way to put it all together to meet the nervous system needs of someone stressed by pain. And none, to my eye, was clearly trauma-informed. Given that pain can cause trauma and that trauma can cause pain, I felt that a trauma-informed focus needed to guide my program.

I then decided to take a new tack in educating myself about yoga for pain, or simple stretching, gentle strengthening, and mindful breathing. I left the yoga books for a time and turned to learning as much as I could about the neuroscience of pain. From my trauma work in teaching yoga to veterans, incarcerated people, refugees, shelter residents, and the diverse group of professionals who worked with them, I had already experienced a body-based yoga program as a strong healing tool. After learning as much as I could about the science of pain, I finally saw my direction.

Key Points to the GreenTREE Yoga® Approach

1. As stated by Neal Pearson, Shelly Prosko, and Marlysa Sullivan in *Yoga and Science in Pain Care* (2019), there is no pain center in the brain. Pain is complex and needs to be addressed in ways that include the interplay of multiple perspectives, including biology, psychology, and physiology.
2. Any pain program involving movement and breathing should be trauma-informed, designed to create a sense of safety, to empower individuals in their own recovery, and to be simple both to teach and to do. Often people in pain are mentally and physically exhausted.
3. The pain program must link breath to movement, empowering individuals to manage their nervous system. Teaching breath awareness and ways to use the breath for self-regulation is not an add-on to a class; rather, breathwork stands as an integral component to any program.
4. As with trauma recovery, pain management programs should be guided by an awareness that the brain can change or rewire.
5. Accessible resources are a valuable program component. Empowering individuals with knowledge and resources can help them feel less trapped by pain:
   a. Simple handouts explaining the benefits of moving and breathing can inspire individuals to practice a few minutes or more a day.
   b. Free audio and videos to practice at home or at work can support any program.

To Recap: This program grew from educating myself on pain, from many years of teaching trauma-informed yoga, and from listening to the feedback from my classes, professional trainings, and national and global summit presentations. It follows the GreenTREE Yoga® Approach: Building Safety, Supporting Empowerment, and Maintaining Simplicity. Developing this whole-body program with a focus on linking simple stretching, gentle strengthening, and mindful breathing was truly an iterative and collaborative process. Although this book provides background information, it is not necessary to do the program—the practice sequences in Part III alone provide a strong starting point. You can then grow your program as meets your personal and professional needs.

Introduction

Let's begin with a revised definition of pain offered by the International Association for the Study of Pain that has been used as a standard since it was first put forth in 1979.[1] It states that pain is: "An unpleasant sensory and emotional experience associated with, or resembling that associated with, actual or potential tissue damage." It adds that: "Pain is always a personal experience that is influenced to varying degrees by biological, psychological, and social factors." We use this definition as a touch point throughout this book. If there was one type of pain and one pain center in the brain, this book might not be necessary. But there are many types of pain, some of which are not fully understood, and there is no pain center in the brain.

This book is guided by an important scientific fact: physical and emotional stress can increase pain and decrease the ability to learn new ways of both managing and perceiving pain. So, a reasonable management strategy is to teach individuals how to reduce their emotional and physical stress levels even while in pain. Instead of focusing on one type of pain, this book offers a whole-body tip-to-toe approach connecting mind, body, and breath. To provide some understanding of pain, and therefore some of the challenges in pain management and treatment, it considers the fascinating science of how pain signals work, how that signaling can change based on what we do and even what we think, how our brain maps are part of the pain mix, and how individuals learn, and can perhaps unlearn, pain.

The book includes accessible background science as an offering to those interested in considering what may be new ideas to frame a pain management strategy. Knowing that there is science behind these yoga practices may then inspire you to use the practice sequences outlined in Part III. Studies have shown that becoming educated about pain can be an important management tool. But again, you do not have to understand or even be interested in learning the current scientific thinking on pain to teach or to practice the simple yoga in this book. You may perhaps practice first and come back later to explore the science.

This book also serves as an easy-to-use, practical manual for people suffering from pain and for those who work with them. Simple strategies can bring relief to the whole person, body and mind, through self-regulation skills and doing simple stretches "in a way that feels comfortable for you today." These stretching, strengthening, and breathing ideas are not presented separately. Rather, the suggested practices range from short breaks to longer practices, and celebrate the yogic idea that the breath is the heart of a practice and not something to be done before or after the yoga poses. There is much to be gained from teaching in a way that empowers people to experience the benefits of pairing simple movement with mindful breathing.

While I will highlight what is covered in the book, perhaps some testimonials from veterans and refugees on this pain management program could set the stage. (See www.greentreeyoga.org/pain-management-resources for the inspiring audio recordings of these comments.)

Comments from Veterans

I can't believe I am saying this, but right now, at this moment, I am not feeling any pain.

The program has helped me reduce my blood pressure by 10–20 points… helped me to heal quickly. It's helped me reduce my pain medication by 20 to 30 percent…

It motivates me to do the movements…like today I was in a lot of pain and very little pain now.

Doing this yoga for pain, I no longer need to get epidurals or shots for my back or anything else.

Comments from Refugee Women

I want to teach my group. Today I feel more comfortable; before I take this class, my body had pain everywhere. When I start this class I feel more relaxing and I try to move every second…

I can teach my kids and my work and every morning I do the stretch.

I am exciting [sic] to share with all the ladies with back pain. We meet every Saturday and do all the exercises we learned at this class. Thank you!

I feel much lighter, like I am up there, not down on the floor.

INTRODUCTION

My back feels so much better; I like the Kitchen Stretch!

I did the stretches and breathing at work when I really hurt. My boss wanted to know what I was doing, so I showed her and she wants to do it too.

After last week's class, I had the best night's sleep. I haven't slept all the way through, the night is so long. It was the best sleep.

I remember what you say, "find a better way to move," at night when I have pain in my legs.

I was just moving my shoulders and moving around... I heard you say, "move when you can, stretch, don't be still."

I had a stroke a while ago, I have a lot of pain. I do this at home and it feels better.

My shoulders were so heavy—now, after the stretching and breathing, my shoulders feel light. I am really surprised.

The women in my group say it works for their back pain, a lot of back pain in my community. They do it at home too.

They would love the booklets so they can do it at home!

CHAPTER SUMMARIES
Part I. The Science of Healing: To Make Whole

Chapter 1: The Basics. To better understand the possibilities for managing and healing pain, it is important to understand how the brain can change. Therefore, a section on neuroplasticity should start the story. Pain signals are processed in and can even be generated by the brain. So the discussion must start with a working understanding of neurons, which are the cells that send and receive these pain signals. Neurons are also the cells that can create changes. This chapter can bring a new understanding of the many options for managing pain. Discussing the various types and causes of pain underscores that pain is a complex subject. Because there are so many types of pain and no one pain center in the brain, it makes sense that a multidisciplinary approach to pain management is becoming more widely researched and accepted.

Chapter 2: Movement. Common medical advice for back pain used to be to move as little as possible, relying on rest and medication. Now there is a strong body of scientific work supporting the idea that appropriate movement can help, not hinder, the healing process. This chapter discusses the importance of movement to increase flexibility, which can reduce muscle spasms and pressure on nerves and joints. Appropriate movement can also increase the range of motion for joints, as it stimulates the synovial membranes and lubricates joints. Movement also provides opportunities to strengthen bones and muscles, especially the core muscles, which are key in stability, balance, and back and joint health. Lastly, but of key importance, science continues to show that moving and exercising can create physiological changes in the body that can improve mood, decrease stress, and improve the ability to learn.

Chapter 3: The Mind–Body Connection. Well into the 20th century, Western medicine continued to embrace the 18th-century philosopher René Descartes' idea of the mind and body being separate entities, that is, man as a machine with the brain in control of the body. These ideas dominated the two main approaches to pain management as many physicians relied on surgery and/or pharmacological treatments. Over time, it has become clear to many in the medical field that opportunities for whole-body healing should be included. That surgery and drugs do not always need to be the first choice or only option represents nothing short of a sea change in medical thinking. The first section looks at the components of this profound shift in thinking about treating pain.

To better understand the link between managing stress and pain, we look at the stress cycle, known as the hypothalamic–pituitary–adrenal (HPA) cycle. This discussion leads directly to polyvagal theory, the seminal work done by Stephen Porges, PhD, lending more insight into the dynamic interplay among stress, the body, and the mind. The logical next point of discussion is that of pain as perception, which means that pain can be as much about what is happening in the mind as about what is happening in the body. But how we think about or perceive pain does not mean that the pain is not real or that "it's all in your head." Rather, it may mean that the perception of pain plays a role both in causing pain and in helping to manage and recover from pain.

The mind–body connection is front-and-center as the role of education about pain, pain perception, and ideas on how to manage pain gains scientific support. An example is the success of studies showing that both mindfulness and cognitive behavioral therapy (CBT) can help reduce pain. What you think matters, which is an empowering thought.

Again, a discussion of the science of breathing can both inform and inspire. Why is the role of the breath in mediating the mind–body connection a key to pain management? How we breathe can directly affect the nervous system and how the brain functions. How we choose to breathe can calm, energize, or even agitate. The last section in this chapter discusses how a body-based yoga practice puts it all together. Yoga can be used to set the stage for and guide neuroplastic changes that support pain management.

Part II. Making It Trauma-Informed: Ideas for Teachers and Healthcare Providers

Chapter 4: What Is a Trauma-Informed Approach and Why Is It Important? Why is there a chapter on trauma in a book on pain management? Science has shown what many already know through common sense and experience. Pain and trauma, both emotional and physical, are intertwined. Pain can cause trauma, and trauma can cause pain. This chapter discusses what trauma-informed means, and why a trauma-informed approach can strengthen pain management programs. If you are using this book to manage your own pain, this chapter can give you insights into the physiological effects of trauma. It can also explain and perhaps validate your responses to situations and teachers. Some basic understanding can inspire you to try these practices as part of your trauma recovery, as a way to take charge of your life.

A trauma-informed approach means your methods are framed by an awareness of how trauma can affect a person and what might be helpful in trauma recovery, although please take special note that trauma-informed does not mean that you need to know someone's specific trauma. This chapter discusses the various components of what makes an approach trauma-informed. How can simple language support verbal communications that are effective and empowering but not overwhelming? How can you empower individuals to build that feeling of safety within their own body? How are you building a feeling of safety in the room? How do you keep someone engaged so they pay attention (something necessary to learn new things) without overwhelming them with too much information? The chapter ends strongly with a section on ways to empower people. As many of the top trauma researchers and authors agree, a key to trauma recovery is a feeling of being in control, something lacking at the time of the trauma, and most probably lacking as someone experiences pain.

This chapter is informed by the science of polyvagal theory. The Green-TREE Yoga® Approach guides this trauma-informed discussion—developing strategies for building a sense of safety, supporting empowerment, and maintaining simplicity—but additionally, providing clear information on the benefits and reasons for practicing these tools can be empowering. Someone can be informed and inspired, choosing to be a participant in their recovery.

Part III. Simple Practices for Everyone: At Home, at Work, or in a Healthcare Setting

Chapters 5–8: The Practice. These chapters are the "how to" of this book. **Chapter 5** provides an introduction and descriptions of the practice sequences. **Chapters 6**, **7**, and **8** include outlines and the practice sequences. These are easy to teach, and as importantly, easy to understand. The sequences can be done anywhere—in a healthcare setting, a cramped room with a dirty carpet, a hospital room, a prison gym, a lovely yoga space, or at someone's home or work. A chair can be useful, but the practice is also adaptable for lying down. No other props are necessary.

The practice sequences range from short breaks to longer practices, creating many options for practicing. Options include standing, seated, kneeling, and lying down, with combinations and variations to meet differing needs and interests. The practice sequences have an easy-to-follow format including key phrases, cueing, and photographs. Some also include MP3s or MP4s, which can be used as teaching tools or to support personal practice. Framed around the seven teaching points of this program (see Chapter 5), these sequences offer many opportunities to set up success. (See www.greentreeyoga.org/pain-management-resources for handouts to support student, client, and patient education.)

Please note: These practices are not medical advice. If you have any questions about your ability to use simple stretching and breathing for pain management, please be advised by a medical professional.

Part IV: Appendices

Appendix A contains photographs of the poses and variations. It is also available to download (www.greentreeyoga.org/pain-management-resources).

Appendix B contains information on the resources that have informed the GreenTREE Yoga® Approach.

PART I
THE SCIENCE OF HEALING
To Make Whole

CHAPTER 1

The Basics

Why Science Basics Can Inform Your Program

Pain is curious. Pain is complicated. Let's explore two examples. The first seems straightforward. Reported in the *British Medical Journal* (*BMJ*), a builder's fall in 1995 resulted in a large nail piercing his boot.[1] In agony, the man was rushed to hospital and heavily sedated. But, on removing the boot, it was discovered that the nail had not penetrated the foot but had actually gone between his toes. Had the man's agony been real? Another example is when a limb (an arm or a leg) or part of a limb is lost through injury or disease. Why can someone then continue to feel pain or other sensations in that absent or phantom limb? A renowned neuroscientist came up with a novel idea to help phantom limb pain, and we will circle back to this later in the chapter.

Again, pain is complicated. Pain has different causes, some of which are poorly understood. Pain has different treatments, some of which are effective, and some of which are not. People can have very different pain experiences based on their genetics, experience, and perceptions about pain. Sometimes pain goes away. Sometimes it gets worse, even though the original source of pain goes away.

Whether you are circling back to this section after exploring the practice sequences in Part III or you have decided to start with the science, welcome. You may want to better understand the types and causes of pain because you suffer from pain or work with those who do. You may know this basic science already, so it's a helpful review, or the science may be new to you. It is offered as a way to frame a pain management strategy. Knowing there is peer-reviewed science behind these ideas may inspire you to experience some of the simple stretching, gentle strengthening, and mindful breathing practices in Part III.

A good place to start this story is at the beginning. The science basics are included in this first chapter because the nervous system, from the building blocks to the signal centers to the processing headquarters, figures front and center in the rest of this book. Moving to both stretch and strengthen, breathing strategies, stress management approaches, and making a pain management plan all comes back to what's happening at the cellular level.

What Is a Neuron?

The building blocks of our nervous system are neurons, nerve cells found in different parts of the body that send and receive electrical and chemical signals. There are about one hundred billion neurons in the brain. A fun neuron fact is that 80 percent of the neurons outside of the brain are found in the gut. (There is more on what that means in Chapter 3.) Okay, so neurons are nerve cells that send and receive signals, which seems like straightforward science, but because all this happens in a living body and not a machine, there is, of course, so much more. Why do neurons send signals? Where do the signals go? Are the signals the same strength? Does one signal affect the other signals? Do the signals change over time? What happens if a neuron is damaged or dies? The answers all affect pain.

Let's take a quick look at the structure and function of a neuron, and then at what can happen when neurons do what neurons do.

Structure

A neuron has several parts: the cell body, in which the DNA and nucleus are found; the dendrites, which receive signals from other neurons; and the axons, which generate signals to other neurons.

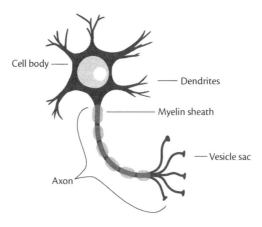

FIGURE 1.1. A NEURON

The axons are covered by myelin sheaths, protective white, fatty insulation that can increase a neuron's signaling speed. At the end of the axons are vesicle sacs, which store and release neurotransmitters. Neurotransmitters are chemical messengers. You may have heard of some of these messengers: dopamine, serotonin, adrenaline (epinephrine), and acetylcholine are examples. These chemical messengers carry signals across synapses, the spaces between the neurons.

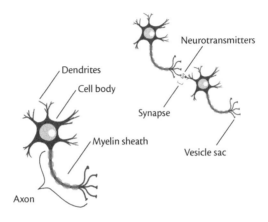

FIGURE I.2. SYNAPSES

Function

There are two types of neurons—sensory and motor. In a healthy system, sensory neurons relay messages from the body to the brain. Motor neurons then send return messages from the brain to the body. But where does that information come from? In a healthy system, the brain receives input, in the form of electrical signals, from two places: the outside environment and the inside environment, that is, the body. You may touch a hot stove. Sensory neurons send that information to the brain where it is processed. Your motor neurons carry immediate signals back to your hand so you can move it. When the burn heals, no more pain signals are sent. Or perhaps you experience lower back pain (sensory signals to the brain), so you change how you stand (motor signals from the brain to the body). This change may take pressure off a spinal nerve root or help strengthen spinal muscles.

Responses may be immediate and instinctive (hand away from stove) or they may be more thoughtful, taking longer to process (changing how you stand). Here is the point at which it gets really interesting. Not only are there different chemical messengers involved in responses, but they do not always do the same thing. Sometimes these neurotransmitters may speed things up, slow things down, or even modulate actions. Science and research are ongoing, and books continue to be written on this important topic.

What Are Glial Cells?
Initially, glial (Greek for glue) cells, which are not neurons, were thought only to be the structural support system for neurons. But ongoing research continues to expand the understanding of the many functions of glial cells. Currently, it is thought that there are about the same number of neurons as glial cells in the brain.[2] Three types of cells make up the glia in the brain: microglia clean up cellular debris from injured areas, acting as macrophages; oligodendrocytes form myelin, the white, fatty coating on the axon of a neuron that can increase signal transmission times; and the most numerous glial cells are the astrocytes, which help maintain cell homeostasis and form part of the blood–brain barrier. Homeostasis is the natural way our body comes back to a state of balance. So how are these glial cells relevant to the pain discussion? We will circle back to what current research is discovering in the discussion on chronic pain later in this chapter.

All Together Now
Individually, neurons are quite interesting. Together, they are fascinating. If you are wondering why there is not a specific pain center in the brain, here is a quick overview of the rest of this chapter. A single neuron fires, which can then activate tens of thousands of other neurons that may then signal others. Neurons can work together in what have been called neural networks or neural circuits. It may not be the most exciting analogy, but thinking of these neural networks as roads can be a useful image. As neuron networks create the roads, signals can go both ways, looping between various parts of the body and the brain. But these large networks of interconnecting neurons are not fixed and operate in a system of self-regulating feedback loops. These complex and ever-changing neural networks help to create our feelings, perceptions, frame of mind, behaviors, and experiences. Neurons create connections based on what we think and what we experience. These thoughts and experiences include the pain we feel and how we think about that pain, which will be discussed later in this chapter and also in Chapter 3.

Let's now consider more of the basics to better understand the science of change.

What Is Neuroplasticity?
Science with a Side of History
To better understand the possibilities for managing and healing pain, it can be helpful to understand that the brain can change. With the ability to image the brain, current neuroscience has found extensive supporting evidence

for what Sigmund Freud, MD, Moshé Feldenkrais, PhD, William James, MD, Ramón y Cajal, MD, and others had discussed for many years. In the late 1800s, William James, often called the father of American psychology, coined the term *plasticity*, which later led to the term *neuroplasticity*, meaning the brain's ability to change. In the 1900s, one of the first Nobel Prizes was won by Ramón y Cajal, who put forth the idea that learning and memory could be changed by strengthening synaptic connections. Again, synapses are the spaces between the neurons across which signals are sent. Then, in 1990, Eric Kandel, MD, won the Nobel Prize for research showing that two things can create conditions for neuroplastic changes: both experience and thought. *The Brain that Changes Itself*, a book by Norman Doidge, MD, provides discussions on how these changes can happen as well as some heartening real-life examples.[3] From this science of change comes a strong sense of possibilities for empowering someone to move away from pain and toward better health. We are, quite simply, not stuck.

"Fire Together, Wire Together"

Neuroplasticity is a process that continues for our lifetime, as long as we receive and process input from the environment and from within ourselves. But the brain does not just change and stay that way, like hardened plastic. David Eagleman, PhD, a Stanford neuroscientist, explains the many possibilities for change in his entertaining and fascinating book, *Livewired: The Inside Story of the Ever-Changing Brain*.[4] Let's look back to 1949, when the researcher Donald Hebb, PhD, published a theory in his book, *The Organization of Behavior*, stating that the synaptic connections strengthen with use.[5] It is how we get better at something. Carla Shatz, PhD, a Stanford neuroscientist, later coined the phrase: "Neurons that fire together, wire together."[6] This concept is important in pain management. It means that pain pathways can strengthen over time, which can increase feelings of pain. It means that ideas about pain and how we respond to pain can become habits. Carla Shatz's corollary idea states that "neurons that fire out of sync, lose their link." Perhaps think about these neuroplastic changes like lifting arm weights. If you are lifting safely, more repetitions can strengthen muscles. What happens if you stop lifting weights? You may see where this idea is going. You lose muscle strength. The common phrase "use it or lose it" is based in neuroscience. Perhaps think about how well you remember skills you have not used since a class you did well in many years ago.

    This science of strengthening and weakening neuronal pathways presents many possibilities for developing pain management strategies. Someone may be able to learn new responses to stress or pain signals. Someone may be able to unlearn certain pain signals. *The Brain's Way of Healing*, another book by Norman Doidge, provides an informative and inspiring discussion chapter on various causes of pain and the brain's ability to heal.[7]

You may be asking if these changes are always for the better. The short answer is that these changes can be adaptive, as when someone learns a new job skill or a new pain management strategy. But changes can be maladaptive, as when someone loses cognitive function or develops chronic pain. A longer answer follows.

What Could Go Wrong?

How is this science relevant to our pain discussion? Neurons are living cells, and how they function, or malfunction, directly affects how we experience pain. Neurons can be damaged from injury, disease, or even toxins. And neurons are part of a bigger system. If we think of neurons as a package delivery system, how many points of disruption can you think of? Is the package damaged? That is, is the neuron able to secrete the appropriate neurotransmitters? In Parkinson's disease, for example, neurons do not secrete enough dopamine, which causes loss of function. Are the dendrites that receive signals from other neurons damaged? Is the neuron dying? Sustained high levels of cortisol, a major stress hormone, can damage the dendrites and eventually cause apoptosis or cell death. Can the neurons repair themselves and sprout new axons to create new and stronger pathways? While certain activities, such as movement and exercise, can support cell repair and health, some physiological and environmental conditions do not. Is the roadway blocked? In multiple sclerosis (MS), the myelin sheath, the covering around the axon, is damaged. The area heals with scarring (sclerosis) that then blocks signal transmissions. The result is a slow loss of function.

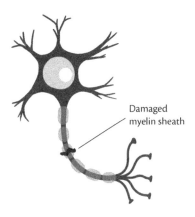

FIGURE 1.3. BLOCKED SIGNALS

There are more questions to consider. Is the roadway damaged or destroyed? Spinal cord injuries are stark examples of such signal interruption. The list of what can go wrong with neurons is not a short one. Other relevant questions are: what happens at the end of the road? Or is it the end of the road? What happens when there is an error, and the signals only go one way? Or what happens when, on that well-traveled road, signals travel too often and to places not on the designated route? The simplistic road image may help as we now turn to the types and some known causes of pain. We come back, again and again, to the fact that pain is complicated.

Types of Pain

Pain can be either acute or chronic. Acute pain stops when the injury heals or when the source of the pain is removed. Chronic pain, for different and some as yet unknown reasons, continues after the initial source of pain stops.

There are a variety of ways to classify pain. Let's consider nociceptive pain and neuropathic pain.

Nociceptive and Neuropathic Pain

Nociceptive Pain: Pain receptors respond to a stimulus. When you stub your toe or walk on a swollen knee, you are experiencing nociceptive pain. In a healthy system, sensory neurons travel from the site of the injury to the brain, which sends motor signals back to stop doing whatever it is that is causing pain. Loren Fishman, MD, and Carol Ardman present a clear discussion in their book, *Yoga for Back Pain*.[8] Nociceptive pain, from the Latin word *nocere*, meaning to harm, happens when sensory signals are transmitted to the brain via sensory receptors called nociceptors. Pain signals from activated nociceptors travel up nerve pathways in the spinal cord, at which point they reach the thalamus, a signal relay station in the midbrain. From there, signals are routed to other parts of the brain for processing and responses. Signals travel at different speeds through various nerve fibers. Two examples are the myelinated (the fatty covering on axons) A-delta fibers traveling at 40 mph (sharp pain) and the unmyelinated C fibers traveling at 3 mph (dull, throbbing pain). Nociceptive pain gets more interesting as pain signals can either be inhibited or strengthened as they travel to the brain. (We will circle back to this idea in the gate theory discussion in Chapter 3.)

Neuropathic Pain: An updated definition of neuropathic pain is: "pain arising as a direct consequence of a lesion or disease affecting the somatosensory system."[9] Somatosensory means conscious sensations or perceptions from pain, pressure, movement, or temperature. The damage can happen without such direct outside stimulus as stubbing a toe. Central neuropathic pain is associated with lesions or damage to nerves (neurons), nerve roots, and nerve pathways in the spinal cord and brain (the central nervous system).[10] As one example, the common condition of sciatica can be caused by spinal bones pressing on the largest nerve in the body, the sciatic nerve, or by inflammation of that nerve from overuse.

Some examples of central neuropathy include spinal cord injuries, shingles, Parkinsonism, MS, traumatic brain injuries (TBIs), and fibromyalgia. Radiculopathy is damage to nerve roots as they exit the spine, which can result from compression of vertebrae on nerves. Examples include spondylolisthesis (one vertebra slips forward over another, commonly caused by arthritis), spondylosis (the fracture of a small area of bone on each side of a vertebra), and spinal stenosis (the narrowing of the spinal canal).[11] Another type is peripheral neuropathic pain, resulting from damage to the nerves located outside the brain and the spinal cord. Symptoms can include numbness, tingling, or weakness in the arms and legs. A common cause of peripheral neuropathic pain, or neuropathy, is diabetes, when nerve fibers are damaged from high levels of glucose in the system. Other peripheral neuropathic pain can result from nerves damaged from chemotherapy or alcohol abuse. Such autoimmune diseases as rheumatoid arthritis, lupus, and fibromyalgia, and viral infections such as Lyme disease, shingles, and Epstein-Barr, can also damage nerves. While scientists are continuing to study the various types of neuropathy and the chronic pain it can create, a top peer-reviewed journal, *The Journal of Neuroscience*, published a study that noted: "The neural mechanisms underlying the development and maintenance of chronic neuropathic pain remain unclear."[12]

Chronic Pain, Learned Pain, and Phantom Pain
So, It's Not All in My Head? Well, yes and no. Pain feels real because it comes from real signals. But in some pain, the signals start in the brain and are sent to the body, which is not the way a healthy system should work. In a healthy system, when an injury heals, the pain goes away. So one source of pain can be a brain-processing issue. What used to be dismissed as psychosomatic pain or someone making it up can be explained as neurons firing with signals that are too strong or that last too long. These errors can create what is called wind-up or chronic pain. One bit of pain can cause a cascading effect in which the brain has learned pain signaling too well, an unfortunate example of "fire together, wire together."

Another area of ongoing research is the role of glial cells. New research looks at glial cells in chronic pain signaling. The way in which neurons and glial cells interact has been identified as a key factor in the development of chronic pain.[13] One issue is that glial cells are able to transmit information through dozens of pathways. R. Douglas Fields, PhD, a glia researcher at the US National Institutes of Health, said that the pain pathways in which the glia operate are "dauntingly complex systems."[14] While acute pain can be a warning sign, chronic pain is not a symptom, as Stanford pain researcher Elliot Krane, MD, puts it, "but its own disease."[15] So, is it all in someone's head? As we continue the discussion, the answer becomes clearer: still yes and no.

There are even more issues complicating the treatment of pain issues. Taking opioid pain medication can cause pain issues. Again, we are back to neurons. Opioid medications work because the body has natural opioid receptor sites. But when flooded with synthetic opioids (medications), the neurons respond by creating more receptor sites. More receptor sites mean the same drug dosage becomes increasingly less effective over time. It is body physiology, not necessarily someone being weak or difficult.

But Nothing Is There: Let's look at a rather striking example of how complex pain issues can be. One of the more interesting examples of the brain sending signals of pain with unquestionably no input from a damaged limb is a condition known as phantom limb. Very simply, someone can feel chronic pain or sensations from a limb that is no longer a part of their body. Scientists who study phantom pain suggest that the upstream signals from the brain still get sent, even though there is no input from downstream, that is, from the missing limb.

V.S. Ramachandran, PhD, a prominent neuroscientist, discusses his research in his intriguing book, *The Tell-Tale Brain: A Neuroscientist's Quest for What Makes Us Human.*[16] He devised a simple and elegant way of treating phantom limb with a mirror box made of materials from a hardware store. Someone places their existing hand in the box divided by a mirror and moves their hand. Because the mirror reverses the image, the brain processes the movement as if it is coming from the missing limb. Many have gotten relief from phantom pain, rewiring their brains by receiving new signals from watching the limb move in the mirror.

Just Refer to the Map: More insights into chronic pain come from looking at brain maps, the areas in the brain that were initially mapped in the 1950s by Wilder Penfield, MD, a neurosurgeon. He called these maps of the body representations the homunculus, which means little man.[17] These brain maps are developed and maintained based on sensory input, that is, from sense receptors in the body feeding information to the brain. And these maps change over time. An idea V.S. Ramachandran offers is that pain signals in one area can expand into another area. Neurons branch out and create new connections sending signals to uninjured areas, resulting in a condition called referred pain. For example, someone may have a shoulder injury, yet they feel pain in their lower back. The exact mechanisms are still being studied.

What Am I Supposed to Do with All of This?

This information is not meant to cause confusion but to give some direction should you want to learn more. As Neal Pearson notes in *Yoga and Science in Pain Care*, science continues to uncover more about the complexity of pain, which underscores the need to have a variety of approaches to pain management.[18] The takeaway point that pain is complicated, and one approach will not serve everyone, is supported in the *Pain Management Best Practices Inter-Agency Task Force Report*.[19] The US Department of Health and Human Services, the US Department of Defense, the US Department of Veterans Affairs, and the Office of National Drug Control Policy convened the Task Force to create findings on acute and chronic pain with regard to the ongoing opioid crisis. This carefully researched report (which is free to download and copy) emphasizes the importance of patient-centered care in both diagnosis and treatment of pain. It gives much useful information on the broad scope of available options, including restorative therapies, medications, behavioral approaches, and complementary and integrative health strategies. Sean Mackey, MD, PhD, from the Stanford University Pain Management Center, echoed these findings: "I'm not pro-opioid. I'm not anti-opioid. I'm pro-patient. There will be no magic bullet, no pill. Chronic pain requires multipronged treatment."[20]

To Recap:

- Neurons are cells that link together to send and receive messages about conditions outside of ourselves and what is going on inside us. Damaged or malfunctioning neurons can be the source of various types of pain.
- A healthy brain can change, a process called neuroplasticity. We are not stuck; we can adapt and learn new ways of responding.
- There are many types and causes of pain. There is not a specific pain center in the brain.
- Pain is complicated.
- Pain is an area of active research. Using what we do now provides many opportunities for crafting and improving new pain management strategies and for improving cellular health.
- It may be of benefit to try various complementary approaches as you educate yourself on pain issues.

CHAPTER 2

Movement

Moving: Why It Matters to Pain Management
Moving in a way that stretches and strengthens muscles can help with pain management. But why? Many wonderful books have been written on the physical and emotional health benefits of movement and exercise. Movement supports cellular repair processes, described by the evolutionary biologist Daniel E. Lieberman, PhD, in *Exercised: Why Something We Never Evolved to Do Is Healthy and Rewarding*.[1] His book presents current studies and ideas on the benefits of exercise, and serves as a strong complement to John Ratey's foundational book, *Spark: The Revolutionary New Science of Exercise and the Brain*.[2] John Ratey discusses the importance of movement and exercise in helping many conditions, including anxiety, depression, addiction, and even attention deficit hyperactivity disorder (ADHD). He presents the science down to the molecular level of positive changes in body physiology that result from movement.

Let's look at how strengthening bones and stretching and strengthening muscles, tendons, and ligaments through movement can provide numerous benefits, including pain relief, increased range of motion (ROM) for joints, increased blood flow (circulation) to facilitate tissue healing, improved immune function, and increased body awareness.

Provides Pain Relief: It may be helpful to keep an image of a healthy spine in good alignment in mind as you read this section.

The muscles and spinal discs maintain the spaces between the bones from which nerves exit. Tight muscles pulling on bones and joints can press on nerves causing pain. Muscle tightness can be the result of postural adaptation (for example, favoring one leg as you walk or using one arm more than the other) or from muscle scarring. Muscles also can become shorter from spasming.[3] The relevant point is that when someone is in pain, they may move less or unevenly. Tight spinal muscles can cause the spinal bones (vertebrae) to press on spinal nerve roots and on spinal discs, causing slipped or bulging discs. Loren Fishman and Carol Ardman note the best way to counteract a muscle spasm that occurs from strain or inflammation is gentle stretching, which includes yoga.[4] Research suggests that 12 months of a consistent stretching program can be as effective as strengthening exercises or manual therapy for someone suffering from chronic neck pain, for example. These consistent stretching programs have also been shown to be an important nonpharmacological treatment (no medication) for low back pain. Studies have also shown that pain sensitivity is reduced by moving in ways that stretch and strengthen muscles.[5,6,7,8,9]

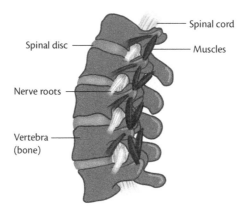

FIGURE 2.1. A HEALTHY SPINE

Improves Range of Motion (ROM): Range of motion is the healthy degree (range) of movement around a joint. Flexibility around joints and good ROM are important for several reasons. Being able to move joints can reduce pain, increase circulation, stimulate the synovial fluid that lubricates joints, and decrease stiffness. Decreased ROM can put extra stress and strain on muscles and other joints as a person moves in uneven ways to compensate for pain or stiffness. For example, walking with more weight on one leg can lead to improper body alignment and increase pain. So good ROM contributes to the balanced stretching and strengthening of muscles and other connective tissues. Maintaining a healthy ROM in large joints (hips and shoulders) can also improve someone's ability to move quickly and safely to keep their balance.

Improves Circulation: Stretching increases movement of blood, synovial fluid (joint fluid), and lymph in the body, which means more exchange of nutrients, fluids, and waste products. This exchange is especially important in areas that have limited or no vasculature (blood vessels). Examples include tendons, ligaments, and spinal discs.

Reduces Inflammation: Studies continue to show that stretching decreases inflammation, highlighting the interactions between the musculoskeletal and immune systems.[10] Daniel Lieberman's book, *Exercised*, presents studies showing that moderate exercise can also reduce inflammation.[11] When muscles remain inactive, inflammation can result. When we move in ways that stretch and strengthen muscles, dozens of messenger proteins that help to control inflammation are secreted. The actions are similar to the wound healing response.[12] Since muscles make up about a third of the human body, it makes sense that keeping active can exert a strong anti-inflammatory effect.

Reduces Stress, Anxiety, and Depression: Stress and anxiety levels have also been identified in factors in back pain.[13,14] Moving in ways that stretch and strengthen muscles can naturally increase levels of serotonin, a neurotransmitter associated with feelings of happiness and well-being.[15,16,17]

Improves Immune Function: As stretching and strengthening movements decrease stress levels, immune function improves.[18] Again, it is body physiology.

Improves Bone Health: Movement that includes weight-bearing and resistance or strengthening exercises can help keep bones healthy. Inactivity, or not moving, can cause loss of bone density. Keep in mind that bone is living tissue. Walking, hiking, and climbing stairs are examples of low-impact activities that can contribute to bone health. Some standing balance yoga poses can provide weight-bearing or resistance exercises.

Builds Body Awareness: Moshé Feldenkrais, PhD, was a brilliant physicist who worked in the Nobel Prize-winning Curie lab on nuclear research. Then he became a renowned teacher, healer, and body-worker. Moshé Feldenkrais developed the program called Awareness Through Movement (ATM), which stresses that awareness comes through small movements made slowly. More simply stated, "Movement is the basis of awareness."[19] Why is this important to pain management strategies? Body awareness is an important tool we can practice. If someone is unaware of how they are feeling or how they are moving, they are less able to use pain management tools that include breathwork, simple stretching, gentle strengthening, and proper alignment.

Moving: How We Do It

How we use our muscles can directly affect how we manage pain. Examples include the muscles surrounding the spine and the dome-shaped muscle under our lungs, the diaphragm. The pain management piece is that we can consciously decide how to use (or misuse) our muscles. Let's start with the types of muscles and how they move.

Three Muscle Types

We have three types of muscles: skeletal, cardiac, and smooth. All three muscle types are similar in four ways: (1) nerves cells (neurons) can excite the muscle cells; (2) muscle cells can contract; (3) muscle cells can extend; and (4) muscle cells are elastic, returning to normal length after stretching or contracting. Skeletal and cardiac muscles are striated. Striated muscles contain tubular structures of myofibrils, which contain the protein filaments of myosin and actin that interact to cause muscle contraction. We can move because skeletal muscles contract or lengthen. As we breathe, the diaphragm, a dome-shaped, skeletal muscle under the lungs, contracts and releases. As cardiac (heart) muscle cells contract and release, blood is pumped to and from the lungs and throughout the body.

Smooth muscles are found in the digestive tract, blood vessels, and other hollow organs. As smooth muscles contract, things get moving: think of the peristaltic contractions in the esophagus as you swallow and in the stomach as you digest food. Smooth muscles are non-striated and contain no myofibrils.

You might want to give yourself 20 seconds to experience the workings of all three types as you read the next few sentences. As is comfortable for you today, run in place or do jumping jacks for about 20 seconds. How are you engaging all three muscle groups? Short answer—you had the thought to move, so your muscles started working to move your bones. Feedback loops of electrical and chemical signals coordinated the movements. Your cardiac muscles started pumping more blood to supply muscles with the necessary molecules to do work, and your arteries and veins started to expand to accommodate the increased blood flow from the heart to the lungs and all around. Keep reading for a gentler experiential muscle opportunity.

How Muscles Move

If you like, as you are reading this sentence, contract the muscles in your legs as if you are trying to lift your kneecaps. Notice the sensations. Then, on your next breath out, release those muscles. You just experienced how your skeletal muscles are under conscious control. But cardiac and smooth muscles are not under conscious voluntary control. They function without you having to think about it. The breathwork exercises in Chapter 6 guide how to control the diaphragm (the dome-shaped muscle under the rib cage). This breathwork becomes a way to manage your heart rate, which controls your blood pressure. It's a stress and pain management tool using conscious muscle control.

Before we take a deeper dive into the science of movement, let's give ourselves a moment of silliness to introduce both the neuromuscular and musculoskeletal systems. Look at a pen and think about moving it. Most would agree that your thoughts alone cannot move the pen. Now look at the pen, think about moving it, and then physically move it. What changed? You moved your hand to the pen because of a chain of electrical and chemical signals from mind to muscles. No such pathways exist between your mind and the pen. Now what if, when you touched the pen, it stuck to your fingers? Sensory touch and sight signals would be sent to your brain, generating a response to shake your hand to release the pen. As an interesting note, brain–computer interface programs are being studied to read electrical signals from thoughts and redirect them around injured muscle pathways to complete signals enabling muscles to move.[20,21]

So how we move and the health of the neurons that allow us to move are central to pain issues. Let's continue with more basics.

The Neuromuscular System

Neuromuscular describes how nerve cells interact with our muscles. Nerves connect to muscles to generate movement. A key fact in understanding pain is that our nervous system controls our muscles. Sensory neurons relay information from both external (exteroception) and internal (interoception) sources to the various parts of the brain. Does something feel warm and fuzzy, or does it feel burning hot? These signals are sorted and routed to other parts of the brain by way of the thalamus. Then a motor neuron response, either conscious or unconscious, happens. Do we want more of something, or do we move away quickly? These motor responses, that is, our muscles moving, come from one or both of these systems: (1) lower motor neurons in the brainstem (instinctive responses) and spinal cord; and (2) upper motor neurons originating in the cerebral cortex (higher-level thinking).[22] The interesting fact about pain is that upper motor neuron signals can override lower motor neuron signals. (We will circle back to what this means for pain perception and management in Chapter 3.) When a muscle fiber receives a signal from the nervous system, myosin filaments are stimulated, pulling actin filaments closer together so a muscle contracts. The specialized synapse between a neuron and the muscle it stimulates is called the neuromuscular junction. In a healthy system, the sensory and motor signals create feedback loops that allow us to fine-tune movements in real-time.

Now let's move ahead and talk more about muscles.

The Musculoskeletal System

The musculoskeletal system includes the skeleton (what the muscles move) and other parts of the body assisting in that movement. Our genetics and our experiences determine how we hold ourselves or how our skeleton aligns. Using, or misusing, muscles reminds me of a quote sometimes attributed to Eldridge Cleaver: "You are either part of the solution or part of the problem." To my mind, thinking of muscles as "part of the solution or part of the problem" provides many opportunities for pain management.

Moving right along, let's look at other areas affected by and that affect the workings of our skeletal muscles.

The Skeleton: Bones are relevant to a pain discussion because bones can press on nerves. Such unhealthy bone conditions as injury or infections can also cause pain. Do you remember how many bones are in the human body? The human body has 206 bones. If you like math—your hands, with 27 bones each, contain what percentage of all our bones? Twenty-five percent. Another number to add to the mix is the 26 bones in each foot. If you are still playing with numbers, what percentage of your bones is in your hands and feet? About 50 percent of the total number, which is a lot of moving parts and a lot of joints. One more number if you like. Imagine a giraffe, specifically the neck, as it stretches toward treetop leaves. You have seven bones in your neck—how many does a giraffe have? Both you and a giraffe have seven neck bones or cervical vertebrae. Our spines have 26 bones: seven in the cervical spine (neck); 12 in the thoracic spine (midback); five in the lumbar spine (the low back); plus the sacrum and coccyx (tailbone).

Joints: Joints are places in the body where bones connect. Healthy joints provide stability and support for those bones. Some joints are stable and do not move, some move a little, and some move a lot. Synarthrosis joints (sutures) connect the skull bones, and after infancy do not move. Amphiarthrosis joints move a little, like our vertebral joints (spine) or the front of the pubic bone. Diarthrosis joints are free moving and include the wrist, elbow, knees, shoulders, and, of course, the hip joints.

These are also called synovial joints because the bones and cartilage are joined with a fibrous joint capsule lined with synovial fluid. When we move, synovial fluid decreases bone friction as parts of the joint move against each other. Synovial joints are the most common joint in the body and have the greatest degree of movement or range of motion. You may hear a popping sound as you stretch, which can be from gases being released from these areas. The bursae are sac-like structures filled with a fluid similar to synovial fluid, reducing friction in a healthy system. Knee, elbow, hip, foot, and shoulder joints contain bursae.

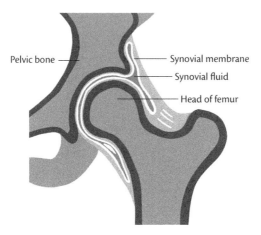

FIGURE 2.2. A HEALTHY HIP JOINT

Skeletal Muscles: There are about 650 skeletal muscles in the human body. To recap, the musculoskeletal system provides support, stability, protection, and movement. Again, this book does not focus on specific muscle groups or areas of pain. Rather, it's a tip-to-toe approach using breathwork, stretching, and strengthening to reduce overall tension in the mind and body.

Major Muscle Groups: It is helpful to consider some of the major muscle groups included in each of this book's practices. The following is one way to group exercises:[23]

1. Arm muscles: triceps (top back of arm), biceps (front top of arm), forearm, shoulder.

2. Core muscles: abdominals and obliques—chest (pectoralis) (front core), trapezius and latissimus dorsi (back core).

3. Lower body: gluteus maximus/medius/minimus (back body), hip flexors (psoas, front).

4. Legs: quadriceps (upper front); hamstrings (upper back), calves (lower back).

5. Chest and back muscles: trapezius, deltoid, rhomboids, latissimus dorsi, erector spinae, pectoralis major, obliques, rectus abdominus.

Fascia: Fascia, from the Latin word *facia*, means band or swath. Fascia is a band of connective tissue that attaches to and stabilizes muscles and internal organs. Fascia connects muscles to other muscles. Deep fascia surrounds individual muscles and is dense with sensory receptors and thin blood vessels. Bands of plantar fascia run across the bottoms of your feet.

Tendons and Ligaments: Both tendons and ligaments are made of dense connective tissue comprised of collagen fiber bundles. Ligaments connect bones to other bones, creating stable joints. Tendons connect muscles and bones, allowing for movement. Synovial fluid lubricates tendons and joints. Fun tendon fact: the largest tendon is the Achilles tendon. Now some fun facts about moving that pen: each hand has over 30 muscles. But you probably only used your fingers, which only have tendons and ligaments. These fibrous bundles have little to no blood supply, so healing fingers can take more time than vascularized muscles, as any rock climber, musician, or someone with a sprained finger can tell you.

Cartilage: Cartilage is another type of connective tissue made from collagen and elastin. There are three types of cartilage in the body: hyaline, elastic, and fibrous. Cartilage has no nerve or vascular connections, so nutrients come from surrounding fluids. Hyaline cartilage is in the larynx and trachea and in the joints where bones touch. Elastic cartilage provides shape and support in the outer ear and epiglottis. Fibrous cartilage is in spinal discs and the pubic symphysis (front of the pubic bone). For this pain discussion, it's worth noting that the three types of cartilage function to reduce skeletal friction and absorb shock in the body.

Spinal Discs: Spinal discs, also called intervertebral spinal discs, are located between the vertebrae, the bones in the spine. With a gel-like center covered in a tougher exterior, spinal discs act as shock absorbers. Moving is one way to keep spinal discs healthy.

Moving: Doing It Better

Most of us move throughout the day. Some people move without giving it much thought. Others move in a more thoughtful way, either because moving is painful, or because they want to derive benefits from their efforts. Most of us want to move in a way that makes us feel better. Let's consider a few ways to make that happen.

Finding *Your* Way

As Moshé Feldenkrais taught, there is not a right way to move; there is a better way to move. Thinking of moving in terms of the right way "has no future development…the 'better' can be improved, the 'right' remains the limit forever."[24] Inspired by his book, *The Elusive Obvious: The Convergence of Movement, Neuroplasticity & Health*, I designed the practice sequences in Part III to meet someone where they are.

Setup for Success: Someone can adapt to their physical and emotional needs for that day. These needs include energy levels as well as pain levels. If they feel they don't have the energy to stretch, you have failed to set them up for success. Unless the medical advice is not to move, avoiding simple stretching may create more pain.

Let the Feeling Be Your Guide: Rather than having an end point in mind—"I need to get my leg here"—give attention to how the stretch is feeling. Bob Anderson's best-selling guide, *Stretching*, offers that "with pain, no gain." He recommends paying attention to the *feel* of what you are doing as you stretch.[25] As Loren Fishman and Carol Ardman advise, any burning, numbness, or tingling means stopping the stretch immediately.[26]

Less Is More: The idea that pain is weakness leaving the body isn't part of this book's pain management plan. The approach of pushing through the pain or overstretching muscles can cause real injury. Body physiology includes a protective mechanism in the muscle cells that sense both degree of stretch and the weight load. Too much stretch or too much weight sends immediate signals to the muscles to tighten. It's a protective mechanism for joints and supporting tissues. Micro-stretching is used to describe stretching to 30–40 percent, with a 100 percent stretch being slightly painful. This form of stretching was shown to be more effective than stretching to the point of pain or discomfort.[27]

Less Is Still More: An effective and dedicated stretching practice does not have to be a large commitment of time. Even several minutes a day can bring benefits.[28]

The Big Picture: To focus a stretch on certain areas, it can be helpful first to stretch above and then below that area. This approach makes sense as a tight area can pull on surrounding areas. This idea is one reason all the practices in this book, which include seating, standing, and lying down postures, begin with Tip-to-Toe Stretch.

Types of Stretching

One way to group stretching techniques includes static, dynamic, PNF (proprioceptive neuromuscular facilitation), and ballistic stretches. In this book's trauma-informed practices, gentle forms of the first three techniques are used.

Static stretching is stretching the muscle to some point of sensation of tension, and holding the stretch for a certain amount of time. Static stretches of about 15–30 seconds can increase range of motion.[29,30,31] *Dynamic stretching* refers to an active stretch, often involving moving to some degree within a joint's range of motion. *Proprioceptive neuromuscular facilitation* is a mouthful but worth teasing apart. Proprioception is sensing where your body is in space. Extending your leg behind you and sensing that your foot is there is an example. In the brain, the posterior cingulate acts like our GPS (see the discussion on the neuromuscular system). Facilitate means to make something easier. Facilitation in physiology means increasing the neurons' synaptic connections in the short term.

Okay, so how do we use some aspects of PNF for our stretching benefit? It involves contracting a muscle or its agonist muscle before stretching. A quick recap—muscles move in pairs: as one contracts, another lengthens. Front and back leg muscles (quadriceps and hamstrings) and front and back arm muscles (biceps and triceps) are examples. Various combinations of holding agonist and antagonist muscle contractions can create the PNF response and increase stretching—1-2-3 Shoulder Stretch and #4 Hip Stretch in Part III use this technique.

Strengthening: Alignment and Core

We identified one benefit of muscle strengthening, which is increased bone density. Let's consider two more ways that strengthening muscles are relevant to this pain discussion: improving alignment and building core muscles. Alignment refers to how it all stacks up—your bones, that is. Building core muscles, the muscles that surround the spine (front and back), makes moving and holding yourself in good alignment easier. While stretching has many benefits, stretching with bad form or poor alignment can cause injuries or aggravate existing injuries.[32] Let's look at both alignment and building core muscles in more detail.

Alignment: Telling someone to stand up straight may be well-intended but misses the mark for maintaining a healthy back. The back has three natural curves that form somewhat of an "S" shape from the side view: the cervical curve of the neck, the thoracic curve of the midback, and the lumbar curve of the low back. These curves are important as shock absorbers for the spine and in keeping the rest of the body in alignment for healthy movement. "Stand up straight!" could more helpfully be: "Chin lifts, shoulders back, hips back a bit." There you have three natural curves of the spine, ready to serve and protect.

Does it matter if while you are recovering from a knee or hip injury you walk around a bit lopsided? Does it matter if you spend many hours a day hunched over a screen? Yes, and yes. Bad posture is misalignment and can amplify pain from extra pressure on nerves and joints. Over time, or owing to injury, the muscles and connective tissue around the spine can lose flexibility and strength. So, as someone does normal activities, perhaps reaching to grab something on a top shelf, twisting to look behind, or bending to pick something up, it is the low back that picks up the slack. It's the lower back that feels the extra stress and strain of the movement. Charlotte Bell's carefully crafted book on hip health is accessible and easy to use. *Hip-Health Asana: The Yoga Practitioners' Guide to Protecting the Hips and Avoiding SI Joint Pain* (2018) provides a clear path forward to hip health and is a valuable addition to anyone's yoga library (see Appendix B for a list of resources).

Core: Remember that core muscles wrap all around the central part of you, meaning front and back. Core muscles provide structure, support, and protection for the spine and internal organs. Core muscles are also involved in arm and leg movement. Studies have shown that strengthening the core is an important part of managing back pain.[33,34,35] Core muscles stretch from your thighs to the bottom of your breastbone and include some major back muscles. Getting a mental image of the wraparound support offered by all these muscles may inspire you as you choose your practices from the practice sequences in Part III.

To Recap:

- Understanding how we move can inspire us to move with more awareness.
- Being more aware can make our pain management strategies more effective.
- Movement and exercises that include stretching, strengthening, and alignment have diverse mental and physical health benefits, some of which are commonly understood, and some of which may be new to you.
- Stretching and strengthening muscles can reduce pain and inflammation by reducing pressure on joints and nerves, increasing circulation to the affected areas, and improving alignment.
- Movement and exercise can change body chemistry in ways that reduce stress and anxiety, making us more able to unlearn some responses and learn new, more adaptive responses.
- Simple, gentle stretches can have much benefit, which is why this book focuses on simple tip-to-toe stretches paired with mindful breathing.

CHAPTER 3

The Mind–Body Connection

The Mind and the Brain

In the last chapter, we looked at how muscles, bones, nerves, and other connective tissue can affect pain. Now let's look more closely at the benefits of considering the communication between the mind and the body in pain management discussions. Let's consider one definition of the mind, put forth by Daniel Siegel, MD, as his way to foster dialogue across disciplines. As he explains in *The Developing Mind: How Relationships and the Brain Interact to Shape Who We Are*: "A core aspect of the mind is an embedded and relational process that regulates the flow of energy and information."[1] Our brain structure begins with our genetics. It then is shaped by our life experiences. This ongoing process continues to influence how the brain receives, processes, and sends information. Daniel Siegel offers a point relevant to our pain discussion: the mind is a process influenced by connections with ourselves and with others. This ever-changing life process means we are not stuck. For those who want more information, Daniel Siegel's books are accessible and informative resources (see Appendix B).

Let's now look at the physical structure of the brain, which is what is processing incoming information. Then we can consider the ways the mind and the body can shape the physical brain. A useful model of the brain that can help us understand how the signals are sent, received, and what happens in between is called the triune brain.

The Triune Brain: The triune brain model was proposed in the 1960s by Paul MacLean, MD, a neuroscientist and psychiatrist. Even at the time he knew it was simplistic. Yet it continues to provide a general model for understanding.[2] The triune brain has three basic brain components: the reptilian, the limbic, and the neocortex.

The reptilian brain controls our most basic survival functions, all of which are below conscious thought. The reptilian brain, also called the lizard brain, is why we don't have to think about taking each breath or why we don't have to tell our heart to beat faster when we run. The limbic system is considered the emotional center, including the place where memories are first encoded. The evolutionary addition of the neocortex, the site of higher-level thinking, appears only in mammals. A fun brain fact is that the neocortex takes up about 30 percent of the brain. Something to keep in mind is that 70 percent of the brain is taken up by instinctive and emotional functions (reptilian and limbic).

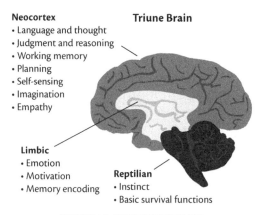

FIGURE 3.1. THE TRIUNE BRAIN

Your Brain on Stress: When we are physically or emotionally stressed, the neocortex functions are overridden by survival or emotional responses. How is that helpful? In stressful situations, quick, reflexive action can protect lives. Taking the time to think it through can be harmful if split-second action is needed. Another brain fact is that it takes longer to process a thought (neocortex) than it does to process a reflexive action (reptilian or limbic). Daniel Kahneman, PhD, a psychologist who won a Nobel Prize in economics, uses this physiological fact to frame his book about decision making: *Thinking Fast and Slow*.[3] He names these response paths System 1 and System 2. System 1 responses are automatic and need little to no conscious effort: dodging a piece of falling debris or pulling someone out of harm's way are examples. Always getting off at the same stop or turning onto the same road are more examples of System 1: things you do automatically, even when deep in thought about something else. Some call this procedural memory. These memories are stored in the nonverbal part of the brain, which allows you to ride a bike or do a dance step without relearning it each time.

If you pause and consider the consequences of sending that text or email, then you have engaged System 2, the high road, higher-level thinking. Making a thoughtful decision takes more time because signals need to travel to the prefrontal cortex. It is body physiology. It takes time to consider if you want to risk injuring your arm to pull someone from harm's way. Another neuroscientist, Joseph Ledoux, PhD, uses the expressions "high road" and "low road" to describe different response times.[4] Some common expressions highlight the difference: "Think before you act;" "Next time count to ten before you answer;" and "He just flew off the handle." Neuroscience explains why taking some time before acting supports making more rational decisions.

> **The Relevant Point:** While this science may be of interest, how is it relevant to pain management? The short answer is that stress management is a key part of pain management. And your ability to manage your stress levels depends on how safe or calm you feel, being consciously aware of feeling stress, and then taking the time to use simple tools to self-regulate. The assessment and response processes integrate the functions of many brain parts. So what? If you want to learn or you want to empower someone else to develop better pain management skills, a key step is learning to pause and think it through before responding. Over time and with practice, a more adaptive response to pain and stress can become a habit. The longer answer pulls together each of the following chapter sections.

Gate Theory

Science, with a Side of History: Another piece of exploring the mind–body connection is a theory that to this day continues to shape the way pain research and treatments are framed. The theory deviated from the simplistic "this–then–that" approach to understanding pain. In 1965, Ronald Melzack, PhD, and Patrick D. Wall, PhD, put forth the gate theory. At the time they said, "No one has ever seen this sort of wiring, but we propose that it's good to look at something like this, given how pain works."[5] Ronald Melzack was a student of Donald Hebb, PhD, and not surprisingly, Ronald Melzack was a pioneer in the study of plasticity in the spinal cord and the brain. While parts of the theory continue to be refined, as Robert Sapolsky, PhD, notes, it continues to inspire many important experiments.[6] Gate theory has advanced how we think about the components of pain experiences. It considers how various pathways are influenced by physical, emotional, and cognitive factors. As Patrick Wall later wrote with regard to the gate theory: "The least, and perhaps the best, that can be said for the 1965 paper is that it provoked discussion and experiment."[7]

Well, What Is It? It's quite a build-up to the question, "What is gate theory?" The short answer is gate theory states that pain impulses can be tamped down or gated in the spinal cord before they even reach the brain for processing a response.

Let's look a bit more at the science of pain signaling before we circle back to practical applications.

Our somatic mechanoreceptors or sensory (afferent) fibers pick up information based on pressure, heat, vibrations, or other mechanical stimulation. These signals travel to the dorsal horn in the spinal cord, which is made up of gray matter.[8] Central transmission cells (T cells) receive signals from both larger, myelinated, and faster fibers (A-beta and A-delta) and smaller, unmyelinated, and slower fibers (C fibers). These cells can either inhibit or excite the sending of signals onward to the brain. The gate theory suggests pain signals can be modulated because the dorsal horn acts as a gate for pain signals. For example, A-beta fibers can create a burst of activity followed by a decrease in activation (think stubbed toe), while C fibers can produce more activation and feed wind-up pain.

It's Complicated: Research continues to show that understanding pain mechanisms is complicated. Let's recap, as these ideas continue to be key in how we think about pain. Neil Pearson notes in his extensive science discussion in *Yoga and Science in Pain Care* that the gate theory explains how pain goes beyond sensory input to include cognitive, emotional, and stress factors.[9] It supports the idea there are various points of entry to managing pain. In other words, science and common sense continue to show that many factors affect pain.

Let's now consider how the science of gate theory supports approaching pain as a phenomenon of perception. This approach allows researchers and practitioners to frame more diverse management strategies.

How We Process Pain: Perception and Emotions

Research continues to show how emotions and our psychological state can affect our physical health. For example, some studies show that stress and anxiety can increase the incidence of back pain.[10,11] At first glance, pain signaling seems a straightforward process: pain (sensory) signals are sent to the brain. Response (motor) signals are sent back to the body. But here is a point at which it gets really interesting. The feeling of pain is also a perception. A perception is how we interpret something based on our senses. That perception can then shape how we interpret that pain. Why does Robert

Sapolsky say, "Pain and the amygdala's response to it is all about context?"[12] The amygdala is part of the limbic system that assesses threat levels. Part of pain processing includes evaluating the meaning of pain and putting that pain in context. We talked about the nail in the boot accident in Chapter 1. A man was in such agony after a nail went through his boot that he had to be heavily sedated. But when the boot was removed, the nail had only gone between his toes. Perception had shaped his quite real and agonizing pain response. The perception of pain is complicated.

Pain and Trauma: Context can be created by emotional states, which raises the interesting connection between pain and trauma. Pain and trauma share some of the same neuronal pathways.[13] Pain and trauma can be physical, emotional, or both. While there is still much to be learned, the pain–trauma connection supports teaching in a trauma-informed way. The pain–trauma connection is so important that the following chapter is devoted to ideas on teaching pain management in a trauma-informed way.

Just a Placebo: You may have heard a dismissive comment that a medication is just a placebo. In Latin, *placebo* means to please. If a placebo helps someone's pain, are they faking the pain or the relief? Researchers tell us that the mind can indeed help to manage pain, something called the belief effect. Multiple studies have found that the placebo or belief effect is real. One study showed that focusing treatments on changing patient belief about pain might provide "substantial and durable pain relief" for people suffering from chronic back pain.[14]

Let's Think It Through: Studies continue to show that cognitive behavioral therapy (CBT) and mindfulness can help people manage pain.[15] CBT is a talk therapy program designed to change maladaptive thought patterns. Being mindful means noticing something in the present. It could be noticing a feeling of pain or discomfort. In that moment of noticing, you have the time to choose a response. For example, do you hold your breath and brace yourself, starting that cascade of stress hormones? Or do you have a ready-to-use one-minute simple stretching or breathing break to lower heart rate, lower blood pressure, and lower muscle tension? Noticing you may want to practice a more adaptive approach is one example of mindfulness. Again, it is body physiology. A quote often attributed to Viktor Frankl, MD, a psychiatrist and survivor of four Nazi concentration camps, is: "Between stimulus and response there is a space. In that space is our power to choose our response. In our response lies our growth and our freedom." Certainly, this idea can be useful in developing a pain management strategy. We will circle back to science-based strategies to help someone create that space that is "our power to choose."

Knowledge Is Power: Why can some general education on pain be helpful? Because being informed can be empowering, which makes it relevant to any pain management discussion. John Kabat-Zinn, PhD, founder of mindfulness-based stress reduction (MBSR), offers that, "If you understand it, you may be able to tolerate it better."[16] In 2018, Nadine Foster and colleagues, for the medical journal *The Lancet*, recommended education and psychological treatment as interventions for chronic low back pain. The recommendation was for these treatments to be done before pharmacological (drug) treatments.[17]

What's in a Name? Terms in recent studies reflect the importance of someone understanding the nature of pain: neurophysiology education (NPE) and pain neuroscience education (PNE) are examples.[18] Several studies examining the nature of pain conclude that pain education had a significant effect on improving quality of life.[19,20] These ideas are why Chapter 2 devotes several sections to exploring some basics about causes and types of pain. Integrating education into pain management strategies inspired the seven teaching points outlined later in Chapter 5. The practice sequences are framed around these educational points, and handouts to share with participants are provided (www.greentreeyoga.org/pain-management-resources).

> **The Synergy Takeaway:** Research continues to support what Neal Pearson states in *Yoga and Science in Pain Care*: "Pain is real. Pain is complex. Pain is not immutable."[21] More healthcare providers are acknowledging the synergy among physical, emotional, and psychological components that feed pain. Again, this awareness is reshaping treatment options. Yet there is still more relevant science to consider as we shape our own accessible and effective pain management strategies.

Stress and the HPA Axis

A Healthy Loop: A strong component of any pain management strategy can be practicing ways to interrupt your stress cycle. You can practice the tools needed to manage and not be controlled by stress. Your stress response starts with the hypothalamic–pituitary–adrenal (HPA) axis.

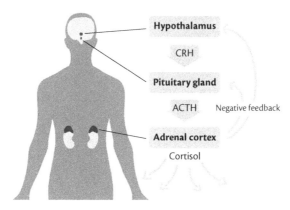

FIGURE 3.2. THE HPA AXIS

It's our stress feedback loop, which, when working in a healthy way, allows us to get amped up for something when we need to be on full alert and ready for action. This same feedback loop brings us back to a calmer state when the danger has passed.

This loop is why neurotransmitters such as adrenaline (epinephrine) and stress hormones such as cortisol can flood our system. In the short term, elevated stress hormone levels can provide positive health benefits such as improved immunity, focus, and energy.

A Loop of Stress: But when our system stays flooded for weeks or even months, the condition becomes chronic stress. Chronic stress is unhealthy for many reasons. Such long-term basic needs as digestion, reproduction, sleeping, immune function, learning, and healing are compromised. Instead of "Well, do you have anything to say about it?" a better question might be "Is there anything you can *do* about it?" And that is the key question because your HPA axis isn't just doing things on its own. Your stress levels result from how you process what is happening, real or perceived events, and then how you respond. Part of building resiliency and pain management skills is managing your stress cycle.

It Should Be Personal: A closer look at how this feedback loop works may inspire you or someone with whom you work to get involved in its management. I think of it as personalizing your stress cycle. In the limbic system or midbrain, various structures receive, filter, relay, and respond to stress signals, again, whether real or perceived stress. The thalamus filters and relays stress signals. Then the amygdala assesses the degree of danger, with input from the hippocampus for context, and sends signals to the hypothalamus. Neurotransmitters and stress hormones are then released, so we can respond. Adrenaline (epinephrine) increases your breathing rate, your heart beats faster, pumping more blood to large muscles, and glucose is released. Then cortisol is secreted to increase energy stores and immune responses. In a healthy system, as the danger passes, the feedback loop then regulates to end the stress response.

The Ebb and Flow of Our Day—Homeostasis: To better appreciate one key automatic body process, consider the term *homeostasis*. Latinized from the Greek words *hómoios* and *stasis*, homeostasis means to stay the same. The term describes biological processes that allow us to come back from extremes, to find a way to keep going in a healthy way. In a healthy system, we perspire when we get hot, cooling us as the moisture evaporates from our skin. We feel thirsty when we get dehydrated, so we grab some water. Homeostasis is why the stress feedback loop in a healthy system resets after the stress has gone. We need to stop sweating, stop drinking water, or stop being on high alert as conditions allow, or negative health effects, and even death, can follow.

Feeding the Loop: But let's back up to consider an important point. How is information on pain, stress, and levels of danger fed into this loop in the first place? We get information from three sources. The first is sensory information from our environment. Is it cold outside? Is that a soft sound? Is that a warm wind? In a process called exteroception, we pick up outside information from our five senses: sight, hearing, touch, smell, and taste. A second source of information comes from sensory signals within us, a process called interoception. Are we thirsty? Is a headache starting? Are we feeling too warm? Stephen Porges offers a third source of cues, which he calls neuroception.[22] Neuroception describes how we pick up cues about safety on a subconscious level. That gut feeling you might feel or sixth sense that makes you shiver may be cues felt and processed in the nonverbal (subcortical) part of the brain. To recap, 80 percent of the neurons found outside the brain are located in the gut. These digestive tract neurons send and receive signals via the vagus nerve to the nonverbal parts of the brain. Perhaps take a moment and consider what this connection means for how our stress levels can affect our digestive system.

Okay, so three information sources feed our HPA axis: sources from the outside, from the inside, and from below the radar. The pain management piece is with increased stress levels, blood pressure increases, and muscles tighten. These physiological changes can also increase pain levels. Increased stress levels over time can also suppress the immune system. Then, over a longer time, autoimmune disorders with painful symptoms can occur. We will circle back to more effects of chronic stress.

Making It More Personal: Two points at which someone could personalize their stress cycle can guide our programs. Again, the first is being aware of feelings of stress or discomfort. The second is to practice and then learn to "give yourself a moment." Give yourself a moment to do what? Giving yourself a moment is not yoga-speak. The idea is to pause, literally. "Oh, this is me being upset. Do I want to be upset or do I want to change how I am feeling?" "The Liberating Power of Mindfulness" is an accessible and inspiring chapter in *The Wise Heart* by Jack Kornfield, PhD.[23] He discusses how a mindful approach can help someone observe their thoughts and then respond in a process that gives them freedom from reactive living. If growing more upset or stressed is not the direction in which the person wants to go, then the second point at which "to personalize your stress response" is to use a management tool. Again, it can be as simple as 1 minute of breathwork, perhaps followed by one minute of a favorite simple stretch (www.greentreeyoga.org/pain-management-resources).

But again, if the HPA loop stays in overdrive because of some damage to the physiological system, the flood of stress hormones can compromise our higher-level thinking abilities. Thinking about and then taking effective action to manage pain becomes much more challenging. Again (and again), because it is a key point, someone can interrupt their stress cycle and build resiliency skills using breathwork and movement. It is body physiology. And it's important to know that there are often ways to regain healthy function in our brains. We are not stuck. It may be inspiring to review the ideas about neuroplasticity in Chapter 1.

Now let's look at the science of breathing that might inspire your trauma-informed strategies for pain management and healing.

The Breath

Notice that sometime in the last few seconds you took a breath in. Was it because you thought, "Oh, I need to breathe in now?" By now you may have breathed out. Was it because you thought, "Okay, now I need to breathe out to rid my body of excess carbon dioxide?" We can get through an entire day, about 20,000 or more breaths, and never once think about breathing because it is an automatic function controlled by the brainstem. A recurring question in this book can be asked again: how does this relate to pain management? Because instead of never giving a second thought to how we breathe, we can use some of those 20,000 breathing opportunities each day. Choosing how we breathe directly affects our heart rate. Therefore, choosing how we breathe directly affects blood pressure and stress levels.[24] And again, stress levels can affect how we think. You may be thinking, "Aha, how I breathe is a way to personalize my stress cycle." You would be correct, but there is more. Breathing is free, it's easy, and it can happen in real-time. Let's talk about the breath. It's nothing short of fascinating.

The Basics of Breathing In: Experiencing how you can manage your breathing may put it front and center in any pain management plan, whether you are teaching breathwork or developing your personal plan. If you like, look at the left side of Figure 3.3 while taking deeper breaths in.

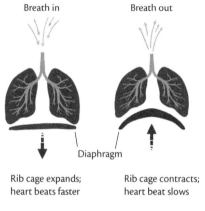

FIGURE 3.3. THE DIAPHRAGM MUSCLE

Envision your lungs expanding because of the negative pressure created as the dome-shaped diaphragm muscle drops, pulling the lungs open. Keep taking longer breaths in, if that is comfortable for you today. Without your body tending toward homeostasis, those longer breaths in may lead to feeling faint. But a signal is being sent, via the vagus nerve (the 10th cranial nerve), from the sinoatrial (SA) node in your heart to the brainstem. That signal is your heart rate is slowing, and therefore your blood pressure is dropping. So the return message from your brain to your heart is to step it up. Now your heart beats faster and harder, maintaining your blood pressure to meet current needs. This science supports the informational cue: "Longer breaths in *can* be energizing." Please note the word *can*, as this breathing can also be agitating for some.

The Basics of Breathing Out: The right side of Figure 3.3 shows the diaphragm muscle moving in a different way. If you like, notice your next breath in. When you are ready, release a long, slow breath out. Envision your diaphragm muscles releasing, like a rubber band sliding back to its original shape. Continue to match your breaths in with longer, slower breaths out, if that is comfortable for you today. This managed breathing is causing a signal to be sent via the vagus nerve from the SA node in your heart to your brainstem. The message is that you don't need as much oxygen now. So a return message from the brainstem to the heart, along the same pathway, is to slow it down. As you are practicing these managed breaths now, your heart rate is slowing, so your blood pressure is dropping. Muscles are also becoming less tight. These changes can happen in real-time with several breaths. This science supports the informational cue: "Longer breaths out *can* lower heart rate, lower blood pressure, and lower muscle tension." Again, please note the word *can*, as while this breathing pattern reduces the heart rate for many, it can be agitating for some.

A Sea of Equanimity: If you like, based only on how it *feels*, take three more breaths with even-length breaths in and out. You are holding steady. Your breathing pattern is not changing your heart rate because no bidirectional signals are being sent between your heart and your brain.

It's Still Personal: How did you do that? Again, in real-time, you thought about how to breathe, so you controlled the diaphragm muscle and started the cycle of your body tending toward homeostasis. Or, quite simply, you chose your breathing pattern.

Tweaking the Physiological Sigh: Let's look at one more useful example. The physiological sigh has been studied for many years. Jack Feldman, PhD, has studied the complex physiology of breathing.[25] He notes the sighing breath we often take naturally every five minutes is essential to maintaining proper lung function. When carbon dioxide levels build up in the blood, we can feel anxious. So a useful breath to practice could be one that quickly lowers those carbon dioxide levels. Instead of just reading about the physiological sigh, you may like to experience it now. Take a deep breath in…then breathe in again on top of that breath in…hold your breath…then sigh the breath out, as deeply as you can. I used the GreenTREE Yoga® Approach to make this breath trauma-informed. You may want to try it one more time if it's comfortable for you today. As you take a deep breath in, stretch your fingers wide…take more breath in and stretch your fingers a bit wider… hold it as long as you like…then, when you are ready, sigh it out, and release your fingers. You now have a quick tool that works in real-time to change how you're feeling. So as not to waste a grounding opportunity, the breath was synced with hand movements. Did you notice the other change? The cue "hold your breath as long as you like" can empower as it builds body awareness. "Am I holding my breath? Am I done holding my breath?" A quick takeaway is it can become a fun exercise for you to make anything more trauma-informed.

A Heartfelt Sigh: What just happened? As you took the deep, double breath in, more alveoli reinflated. Alveoli are the half-a-billion sacs in your lungs from which oxygen enters and carbon dioxide leaves the bloodstream. While you were holding your breath "as long as you like," more carbon dioxide in the blood passed from the capillaries into these sacs. On your long sigh out, carbon dioxide was expelled from your lungs. With this new information, you may like to now envision your sigh facilitating this exchange of gases as you practice the physiological sigh one more time. As you take a deep breath in, stretch your fingers wide...take more breath in and stretch your fingers a bit wider...hold it as long as you like...then, when you are ready, sigh it out, and release your fingers. Breath management in action.

How important are these sighing breaths? Today, ventilators mimic this breathing pattern. Early breathing devices did not, and many patients died.[26] Two or three of these breaths can become an easy tool for someone to decrease feelings of anxiety. You may have noticed that we tend to sigh more when we are upset. Researchers are trying to pinpoint the neurological reasons. Could it be the body's way of tending toward homeostasis?

The Breathing Brain Bonus: If you find the science of breathing fascinating, here is a bit more science to inform and to inspire. Andrew Huberman, PhD, a researcher at Stanford School of Medicine, presents several science-based webinars on the topic.[27] He provides accessible background science to explain why breathwork is a key tool in self-regulation. Again (and again), this science is relevant to pain management, as breathwork offers a key tool in pain management strategies.

The Mechanics of Breathing: Mechanical factors and chemical conditions affect how we breathe. We discussed the importance of the diaphragm muscle in the mechanics of breathing. This key muscle is innervated (stimulated) by the phrenic nerve, a bidirectional nerve that carries both sensory and motor signals. The ancient Greek word *phren* or *phrenos* means diaphragm or mind. Other muscles involved in breathing are the intercostals, which are between the ribs. Take a deep breath now, if that is comfortable, and notice as your shoulders lift. This happens as the intercostals tighten and pull the rib cage up. You may be thinking that simple stretching could create more space for your lungs as you manage your breath. You would be correct.

We spent the first chapter on the basics of neurons because these cells send and receive messages, including pain signals, around and between the brain and the body. Let's look at the signaling that occurs via the phrenic nerve. Jack Feldman and colleagues identified a brainstem region (the pre-Bötzinger complex) that generates rhythmic breathing in mammals.[28] As you have been reading, you may have been breathing in and breathing out without thinking about it. This automatic rhythmic breathing comes from this brainstem region. You have natural rhythm. You breathe and your heart beats in a natural rhythm. What changes if you breathe in, then pause long enough to notice the pause, and then breathe out? What changes if you are breathing as you are talking to someone? The signaling path now travels from the brain's parafacial nucleus. These are signals sent during the physiological sigh or any breathwork in which we consciously manage our breath. If you take a natural breath in but follow it with a deep, forced breath out, you are using both sets of signaling. This is interesting breath science as we consider the many possibilities for breathwork. But there is so much more than breathing mechanics to consider, as we are living organisms, and not machines.

The Chemistry of Breathing: Let's shift to the chemical aspect of breathing. Most of us know that our cells need oxygen to live. But we also need carbon dioxide—it's not just a waste byproduct we breathe out. Much like stress, it's not simply a good/bad designation. "Oxygen good, carbon dioxide bad" does not capture the wonder of what is happening as we breathe. Carbon dioxide in the blood creates carbonic acid (H_2CO_3). If there were a drumroll, here would be a good place. Your body needs this chemical condition in order to release oxygen from the hemoglobin to which it is bound. Healthy breathing is about keeping oxygen and carbon dioxide levels in balance. Breathing is a way to achieve a balance, to bring you back to homeostasis. Andrew Huberman highlights a key sentence in a study that most of us would never find. He quotes the researchers, Balestrino and Somjen: "The brain, by regulating breathing, controls its own excitability."[29] Simply put, this means that how you are feeling, thinking, and responding can be regulated by how you breathe. It's quite an empowering thought. Let's look at two common examples of how breathing affects how someone feels.

Over-breathing happens when someone breathes more quickly or more deeply than normal (hyperventilation). This can lead to a *drop* in carbon dioxide levels in the blood. This breathing pattern can cause feelings of lightheadedness, shortness of breath, or confusion. It can also cause the heart to pound. Feelings of anxiety, stress, or a panic attack can cause "over"-breathing. As mentioned, the body needs carbon dioxide (carbonic acid in the bloodstream) to release oxygen from the hemoglobin. Fun fact: breathing into a paper bag when hyperventilating is rebreathing some carbon dioxide and restoring some oxygen/carbon dioxide balance in the body.

Under-breathing happens when someone's breathing is too shallow or too slow. It can lead to an *increase* in carbon dioxide levels in the blood (hypoventilation). The body's need for oxygen is not met, which can lead to feelings of shortness of breath, anxiety, fatigue, or headaches. Over time, hypoventilation becomes a serious medical condition. Some drug (opioid) overdoses cause hypoventilation.

> **Quick Takeaway:** Please note that someone should consult a medical professional if there are questions about any breathing concerns. Breathing tools are available to decrease stress and anxiety, which can help someone feel calmer and safer. I highly recommend Dr. Huberman's webinars[30] for more on how you can use your breath to better manage your stress levels and improve learning.

Polyvagal Theory

The next step is to consider why that sense of safety is important in any pain management plan. Polyvagal theory (PVT) provides important insights as we shape our plan. Stephen Porges first presented it in 1994.[31] He expanded on the older idea that our autonomic nervous system has two parts that operate automatically. One part is the sympathetic nervous system, often called fight-or-flight. This system is balanced by the parasympathetic system, or rest-and-digest. The nervous system used to be thought of as an on/off or hot/cold system. Signals travel between the body and the brain via the vagus nerve or the 10th cranial nerve, which Charles Darwin called the pneumogastric nerve. Stephen Porges discusses how these bidirectional signals create the brain–heart connection. You may have experienced this connection in the previous breathing opportunity (see Figure 3.3). As shown in Figure 3.4, it is the vagus nerve along which signals travel from the body, including the gut, to the brain.

These vagal connections also affect the larynx, which contains the vocal cords, and the facial muscles. Let's look at what this means for practicing tools for self-regulation and building resiliency skills.

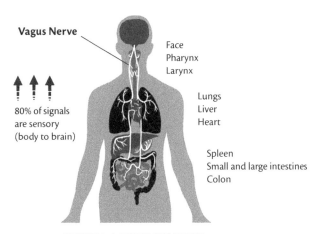

FIGURE 3.4. THE VAGUS NERVE

The Layering Effect: Stephen Porges proposed that in mammals there is a third tier to the nervous system, the social engagement system.[32] Mammals (and that includes us) can override the other two systems by processing cues from other mammals and activating the social engagement system. This vagal brake is an important piece of self-regulation skills, or what some call toning the vagal nerve. Think about a situation in which you want to comfort someone. You might use language. But it's not just your words that offer comfort. It can also be how you sound, that is, your tone of voice, what you emphasize, and how fast you are speaking (all qualities of prosody). But it's not just your words and how you sound. Think about body language and your facial expressions. Would it be a comfort if your gestures and your face relayed feelings of anger or fear? So, as mammals, we can detect various safety cues from voices, growls, or coos. And to review, these sounds reflect the physiological state (responses to how they are *feeling*) of the person or other mammal producing them.

Building Safety: Okay, now let's follow the pain management thread. Empowering someone to build a feeling of safety by accessing their social engagement system and other simple tools to self-regulate can serve as a strong foundation for any pain management strategy. Why should we care about the science of safety and learning? Quite simply, how safe we feel impacts how primed we are for learning. How safe we feel impacts the self-regulation skills we can experience and then learn from the stretching, strengthening, and breathwork of yoga. It is, again and again, body physiology.

Before we continue, it's worth mentioning that for those interested in an accessible and engaging overview of polyvagal theory, *The Pocket Guide* to the Polyvagal Theory: The Transformative Power of Feeling Safe* by Stephen Porges may be a great addition to your library (see Appendix B). Polyvagal theory is referenced in the books of many key researchers and practitioners, including Bessel van der Kolk, MD, Pat Ogden, PhD, Peter Levine, PhD, Daniel Siegel, MD, and Elizabeth Stanley, PhD. A recurring theme is the primary importance in mental and physical health of building feelings of safety. Let's end this chapter by considering how feelings of safety set the stage for learning.

To Learn and to Unlearn

To review a few key points, learning new responses to pain can be an important piece of managing pain. One example is learning a new way to respond when feeling some emotional or physical discomfort. An automatic response might be clenching muscles or holding your breath. Both can set your body's stress cycle in motion and increase pain levels. Let's look at ways to move toward more adaptive and thoughtful responses—perhaps some gentle movements or one minute of mindful breathing. With the thought that how we learn and how we respond are both rooted in body physiology, let's consider a few basic questions.

What Is Learning? Learning is neuroplasticity in action. Think of a child learning math facts, playing an instrument, or hitting a ball. Each skill improves with repetition. The expression "practice makes perfect" is based on neuroscience, as discussed in Chapter 1. Nobel Prizes have been won identifying that neuronal connections (synapses) are strengthened, that is, that we learn something better, through both thought and experience.

What Supports Learning? Parents and teachers have long said, "Pay attention!" Before tossing this idea aside as a "duh" moment, let's look at the science. As we pay attention or focus, certain neurotransmitters (acetylcholine is one) are secreted. Research shows that acetylcholine levels increase as we move, which is yet another reason that school recess and short stretching breaks are important. This increase supports learning (synaptic plasticity and memory formations).[33,34] That gets things started as other neurotransmitters (dopamine is one) take it from there. You may be familiar with the learning challenges of someone with attention deficit disorder (ADD), a condition that includes a dopamine deficiency. If this intrigues you, books continue to be written that take a deep dive into many key neurotransmitters affecting physical, mental, and emotional health (see Appendix B). But for our purposes, it is enough to know that to learn new things, you really do need to be paying attention. Again, short-term stress can help us focus and learn because of the neurotransmitters that are secreted. We need to pay attention to that lion or to traffic or to pain to avoid injury or further pain. Then we need to remember it, which involves memory encoding in the hippocampus. Short-term elevated levels of stress hormones help encode those memories of danger more strongly. Again, it is body physiology.

What Inhibits Learning? Here is where the stress loop (the HPA axis) reenters the conversation. Long periods of stress can inhibit learning. Consider how poorly primed for learning you might be if you did not have enough food, get enough sleep, or feel safe. Studies show that long-term stress can inhibit the formation of new memories (learning), and over time it can kill neurons in the part of the brain that first encodes memories, the hippocampus.[35,36,37] Interesting books continue to be written on stress and memory for those who want to learn more (see Appendix B).

How Do We Unlearn Something? How do you unlearn a response or a habit and learn a new, more adaptive response or habit? The question becomes even more interesting when someone did not consciously learn the response in the first place. As discussed in Chapter 1, chronic pain has been called learned pain or wind-up pain. The source of pain may be gone, but pain signals still get sent because the neuronal pathways have grown stronger.

Even if not all the mechanisms of pain are understood, we can still work with what we do know and what we have observed to be helpful in pain management. One inspiring example of the possibilities for unlearning pain is presented in *The Brain's Way of Healing* by Norman Doidge, MD. He devotes a chapter to the case of Michael Moskowitz, MD, a pain doctor and founder of a pain clinic in California to treat patients who have run out of treatment options.[38] Michael Moskowitz suffered from chronic pain from an injury for over ten years. What did he do? He read 15,000 pages on neuroplasticity. He cured himself, using brain map visualization and various techniques to decrease stress levels while still experiencing pain. The gist of his strategy was that *whenever* he felt pain, he visualized the brain map of the area in which the pain was occurring, and then made himself think of something else that used the same brain area. Why? He wanted to weaken the pain pathways and strengthen more adaptive pathways. Not quick and not easy, but it worked for Michael Moskowitz and patients at his clinic. I highly recommend reading the chapter for a sense of possibilities and inspiration.

Michael Moskowitz's story inspired the Noticing Breath, which gives some practical guidance to the too general suggestion, "Just breathe through it." You continue to notice the area of pain or discomfort on both the breath in and the long, slow breath out. Clenching the muscles and holding the breath are replaced by simple actions that can lower the heart rate, lower blood pressure, and lower muscle tension. It's not a one-time cure, but something to practice to begin rewiring the brain for a new pain response.

> **What's the Takeaway?** How are stress and learning and the HPA axis relevant to pain? Let's recap this important point. Pain can cause stress. Stress interferes with learning. If someone is so stressed that learning new things is a challenge, the first step can be to create strategies to use in real-time that empower someone to lower their stress levels. Hopefully, you are thinking that a short stretching and breathing break would be an easy tool. You would be right. Over time, using this new pain response can weaken the learned, stressful response, a way to put the expression use it or lose it to good use. Someone can choose to change a response and over time create a new habit.

You may see how these ideas are coming together: teaching someone to self-regulate and to learn more adaptive responses is supported by strategies based on safety, empowerment, and simplicity. These ideas are the core of the GreenTREE Yoga® Approach, as outlined later, in Chapter 4. Now let's look at how yoga, which means yoking or union, puts it all together.

How Yoga Puts It All Together: Mind, Body, and Breath

Yoga is both an art and a science, based on thousands of years of thought, practice, and empirical data. Yoga is not a religion but rather an approach to connect mind, body, and spirit or breath. Interestingly, in some cultures the word for breath, life force, or spirit is denoted by the same word: *Qi* or *chi* in Chinese, *pneuma* in ancient Greek, *ruach* in Hebrew, and *prana* in Sanskrit. There are many types of yoga, some more physical and some more focused on breath and spirit. In this book, the simple body-based yoga practices are true to the yogic intention of yoking breath, mind, and body.

Let's review this chapter's key points in a yoga context. Loren Fishman and Carol Ardman note in their book, *Yoga for Back Pain*, that yoga can help reduce pain in significant ways: stretching muscles, strengthening muscles and bones, increasing range of motion, increasing focus and self-awareness, and producing calm.[39] How can yoga support this long and varied list of benefits? It can, because yoga offers both a top-down and bottom-up approach to managing pain.

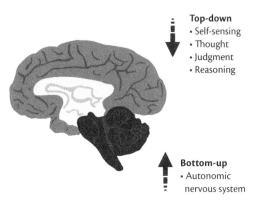

FIGURE 3.5. TOP-DOWN AND BOTTOM-UP

Top-down processing refers to how we process information based on our experiences, expectations, and knowledge.[40] Bottom-up processing refers to the sensory signals the body sends to the brain.

The Mind: Top-down responses are generated from the brain areas involved in higher-level thinking and self-sensing, the neocortex. Several points are relevant to the pain management thread. Let's start with the self-sensing that occurs in the insula and the medial prefrontal cortex. Again, noticing or sensing how you are feeling is a beginning step toward taking effective action to self-regulate. The best-selling author and Director of Research at the Brown University Mindfulness Center, Judson Brewer, MD, PhD, notes in his research that to break the anxiety cycle we need to be *aware* of two things: that we are feeling anxious or panicky, and what then results if we continue.[41] Peer-reviewed studies continue to show yoga can reactivate self-sensing parts of the brain.[42,43] Bessel van der Kolk reminds us that a sense of agency (feeling in control of yourself) begins with interoception, the self-sensing ability: "The greater the awareness, the greater the potential to control our lives."[44]

Talk therapy or mindfulness practices are also processed in the thinking part of the brain (neocortex). To review, these areas function better when someone is not experiencing chronic stress. A third point, as discussed, is that someone needs to be paying attention to learn new things. These varied neocortical functions allow someone to take the time and choose to practice one of their pain management strategies, whether a mindfulness visualization (a top-down approach), or some breathwork linking breath and movement, which brings us to bottom-up strategies.

The Body: Science tells us that 80 percent of nerve fibers are sensory (afferent) and run from the *body* to the brain via the vagus nerve.[45] Bessel van der Kolk notes that this fact provides many opportunities to use the body to calm the nervous system.[46] When trauma and pain co-occur, many top trauma therapists offer that talk therapies and meditation may not be the appropriate place to begin. A more somatically or body-based approach can be a more effective starting point, as both Pat Ogden, PhD, and Peter Levine, PhD, teach in their programs. Pat Ogden's Sensorimotor Psychotherapy® program teaches clinicians how to "read the body." What does that mean? It means that in some therapeutic circles there has been a major shift away from the dominance of talk therapy to the "dominance of nonverbal, body-based, implicit processes over verbal, linguistic, explicit processes."[47] Again, what does that mean? Recognizing that trauma is held in the body means that just talking about something may not be enough. Talking about something (top-down) may not calm someone who is not using verbal parts of the brain: "Insight does not quiet the limbic."[48] Bessel van der Kolk means that talking (top-down) does not calm the emotions (the limbic). The takeaway point for pain management is that the body has proven to be an effective component in learning self-regulation skills. (The many benefits of stretching and strengthening body-based practices, which include yoga, are discussed in Chapter 2.) Breathing, which is also a form of movement, merits its own discussion.

The Breath: How we choose to breathe is a key to bottom-up regulation. We have discussed the science of breathing and included an experiential opportunity. It may be worth revisiting the section; as T.K.V. Desikachar says in *The Heart of Yoga*: "The breath should be your teacher."[49] Being aware of how we breathe is a way to ground in the present, which means being aware that this time is now. Placing both hands over your heart, feeling your heart beating, feeling the rhythm of your breath in and your breath out, can only be done in the present. "I didn't even know I wasn't breathing until we did that hand thing" is a common observation I hear (see Chapter 6). From the simple breath awareness that yoga teaches, someone can choose to take longer breaths out. Someone can take an action in real-time to lower heart rate, blood pressure, and muscle tension. It is body physiology.

Polyvagal Theory Revisited: Here is a quick recap of the role of the breath in polyvagal theory. Stephen Porges explains that breathing gates the influence of the vagus nerve on the heart. We breathe in and our heart rate increases because the influence of the vagus nerve is lessened. As we breathe out, the influence of the vagus is increased and our heart rate decreases.[50] It is the body physiology behind "Just breathe...take some deep breaths out." Be confident that how you choose to breathe or to teach breathwork options can increase health benefits. To repeat, the breath is a free and natural tool, always available to work in real-time. Yoga is a tool that also uses this bottom-up approach to self-regulation.

Mind, Body, and Breath: There is a body of peer-reviewed science that supports practicing yoga to reduce pain, to reduce the biomarkers of stress (cortisol, adrenaline), and to activate the self-sensing parts of the brain.[51,52] One study published in *Cerebral Cortex* found that a regular yoga practice improves pain tolerance by teaching new ways to handle sensory inputs and the emotional responses that come with them, both of which led to changes in activity in the insula, a self-sensing part of the brain.[53] The US Department of Health and Human Services 2019 *Report on Pain Management Best Practices* concluded that "Yoga's use of stretching, breathing, and meditation has also been therapeutic in the treatment of various chronic pain conditions, especially low-back pain."[54] Many peer-reviewed studies in scientific journals continue to show that yoga practices can decrease pain and improve function in adults with chronic lower back pain.[55,56,57,58,59,60,61] Positive results for chronic neck pain treatment and breast cancer survivors have also been reported.[62]

Yoga and Neuroplastic Changes: We have discussed how the process of learning is a process of neuroplastic change. So how someone increases opportunities for learning and unlearning can be an important pain management tool. Michael Merzenich, PhD, a leading expert in the field of neuroplasticity, has written an intriguing book called *Soft-Wired: How the New Science of Brain Plasticity Can Change Your Life.* It is interesting to note that he identifies simple fixes for brain plasticity: "As you move, focus on the feeling of the flow of that movement."[63] To my mind, a body-based yoga practice meets his suggestions. Others include: "Move with your whole body, you have a flexible core and a spine, use them."[64] He advises avoiding stereotypical movements, by which he means the person should explore new ways to move. Michael Merzenich is a world-renowned neuroscientist and does not refer specifically to yoga—his discussions center on how to approach movement. He continues that we need to consciously remind ourselves that we have a whole body "made up of parts that work best when they work together."[65] And perhaps his most inspiring comment is that we are losing major opportunities for improving the health of our brains by exercising in "ways that disengage your brain from participation."[66] In other words, distracting yourself (not paying attention) while moving or exercising may decrease the brain's ability for neuroplastic change.

Part III of this book presents practice sequences designed to link breath with movement and to build body awareness. We move from tip-to-toe to use the whole body and to encourage finding new ways to move. In other words, these body-based yoga sequences are designed to support the neuroplastic changes necessary to creating meaningful pain management strategies that use both top-down and bottom-up processes.

> **To Recap:**
> - Levels of pain, both emotional and physical, are affected by perception, emotions, and stress factors.
> - Someone can personalize their stress cycle using the tools of breath and movement.
> - Pain can cause stress. Stress interferes with learning new strategies for managing pain.
> - Yoga can reduce stress levels and support learning new responses to pain.
> - A body-based yoga practice puts it all together by connecting the mind, the body, and the breath.
> - Yoga combines a top-down and bottom-up approach to reactivate the self-sensing parts of the brain by using body movements and sensations paired with breathwork.
> - Body-based yoga supports neuroplastic changes in the brain.

PART II

MAKING IT TRAUMA-INFORMED

Ideas for Teachers and Healthcare Providers

CHAPTER 4

What Is a Trauma-Informed Approach and Why Is It Important?

This chapter supports my mantra: Be informed and be inspired. Some of these ideas may be new to you; some may serve as a reminder. Either way, the information can help shape a stronger program.

For Your Personal Pain Management Plan: You may be using ideas in this book to manage your own pain, either emotional or physical, or both. While this chapter is written for those who teach, it may be helpful to you for two reasons. One is that understanding some of the physiological effects of trauma can validate that your feelings or responses are not unusual or abnormal. If you feel uneasy or unsafe in a class, you should leave. Be confident that having trauma-informed in a class name does not make it so. You need to be the judge based on how you *feel*. The second reason is that understanding a bit more about trauma can help you find a teacher or class that makes you feel better than when you started the class. It is that simple. Do I feel better than I did an hour ago? Again, you should not *feel* uncomfortable in a class.

Be Informed and Be Inspired: Why is there a chapter on trauma in a book on pain management? To recap, the first reason is that pain can cause trauma, and trauma can cause pain. As discussed, emotional and physical pain are linked because there are shared neuronal pathways.[1,2] The second reason is trauma recovery and pain management strategies share key goals: lowering stress levels, building a sense of safety, and learning self-regulation tools. Therefore, a trauma-informed approach can strengthen a pain management program. It can also build personal resiliency as these skills are practiced. As previously noted, the GreenTREE Yoga® pain management program grew from an established trauma-informed yoga program for those with clinical diagnoses of post-traumatic stress disorder (PTSD) and sexual assault survivors. Most participants also suffered from emotional and physical pain.

A trauma-informed approach means your methods are guided by an awareness of how trauma can affect someone, both emotionally and physically, and what strategies are helpful in trauma recovery. However, trauma-informed does not mean you need to know someone's specific trauma. As discussed in Chapter 3, many top therapists, including Pat Ogden, PhD, Peter Levine, PhD, and Bessel van der Kolk, MD, note that a person may not want to talk about the trauma. They may also not be able to put the trauma or their feelings (alexithymia) into words. As Pat Ogden says, trauma recovery can still happen "using the body as an entry point to the emotions."[3] Peter Levine notes that "a very important fact is that you do not have to consciously remember an event to heal from it."[4] Also consider that asking someone to self-identify as having had trauma is not only inappropriate but can also be quite stressful. Asking someone to name their trauma or potential triggers can turn a group into a triggering situation of over-sharing. The important point is that you can be confident that you can share the benefits of yoga without knowing individual trauma details.

The GreenTREE Yoga® Approach: Well, if you aren't informed about someone's trauma, what then? Three trauma-informed intentions frame this approach: building a sense of safety, supporting empowerment, and maintaining simplicity. These intentions mean that both *what* you choose to teach and *how* you choose to teach hold great importance.

Safety: Building a sense of safety is key, as Stephen Porges' work on polyvagal theory continues to explain with clear science. In a book section titled "Cues of Safety Are the Treatment," he states, "Polyvagal Theory proposes that cues of safety are an efficient and profound antidote for trauma."[5] Judith Herman, MD, a foundational trauma researcher and author, notes in her seminal book, *Trauma and Recovery*, that a sense of safety needs to begin with someone feeling safe in their own body, and growing that to feeling safe in the environment.[6]

Empowerment: A trauma-informed approach empowers someone to feel safe enough to notice how they are feeling. If they are disconnected from their emotions or bodily sensations (dissociation), they are not noticing feelings of stress. If someone is hijacked by feelings of danger (real or perceived), survival functions take over. To review, pausing to notice empowers someone to have the time to choose a more adaptive response. They are, in fact, self-regulating, which means managing their nervous system or autonomic responses. Many therapists agree that empowering a person to feel in control is key. As Judith Herman also said, "The first principle of trauma recovery is the empowerment of the survivor."[7]

Simplicity: Teaching with simplicity has nothing to do with someone's level of intelligence and everything to do with the physiological effects of sustained stress. Stress and pain can also be physically and mentally exhausting. Set yourself up for success sharing yoga by using simple language, simple body movements, and simple breathing exercises. A useful reminder is: More is not better; more is confusing.

Let's look at how you can weave the themes of safety, empowerment, and simplicity into a strong, trauma-informed pain management program.

Language

As friends, teachers, and healthcare providers know, we rely on talking to help. Again (and again), the point to keep front and center in your trauma-informed mind is that someone who is stressed, either from pain or from trauma, may not be fully using the language part of their brain. They probably are not trying to be difficult or resistant. The cascade of stress hormones changes signaling in the brain. The takeaway suggestion is to choose your words carefully. Rather than just talking on and on and hoping that something hits home, consider a few simple guidelines. You may want to reframe your role to that of a guide, not a cruise director. You may find that empowering someone to find what they need today actually takes the pressure off you.

Be Invitational: A few key phrases I learned from *Overcoming Trauma Through Yoga* can set the tone. "If you like..." and "When you are ready..." can often be used.[8] Invitational words are not directive. "Close your eyes" is directive; "Eyes open, eyes closed, your choice" is invitational. To build more safety, I add, "I keep my eyes open so I can let you know when someone joins us."

Avoid Trigger Words and Phrasing: Some phrases can be triggers to those in trauma recovery. Such phrases may sound directive to anyone. You can probably add to this list: "Just relax," "You will like this," "You are safe," or "You need to do this when you feel upset."

Avoid Negative Phrasing: Perhaps consider the feeling evoked when someone says, "Well, if you can't do it this way, then just..." Consider saying:

"It may be more comfortable to put your hands above your knees today. Different days, different stretches." A simple choice replaces a negative word. This simple act of choosing can help build body awareness. Someone may think, "Is this way more comfortable? Maybe I will try it with my hands here." Sometimes we teach without much thought because it's the way we've heard it for years. My suggestion is if you cannot think of positive wording, you might want to keep thinking.

It's All in a Name: Speaking of words, here are some suggestions on naming your classes. Sometimes yoga conjures images of the young and slim in poses of extreme twists or strength. I use simple words to convey the essence of my class: Simple Stretching and Breathing for Pain Management. The phrase trauma-informed could also be off-putting. You know your groups, but as with all things trauma-informed, choose your words thoughtfully.

Avoid Sanskrit Words: Hearing familiar words allows someone to, quite literally, give it a rest. The "it" is the language part of the brain. Using Sanskrit or unfamiliar words can be distracting. Someone may wonder if yoga is a cult or a religion, or what is it anyway with all those odd words? Using a common name for a pose or a breath also offers someone a consistent and easy reference.

Trust the Yoga: I use this phrase when teaching workshops, and people continue to refer to it in follow-up texts and emails, commenting on how trust the yoga guides them in challenging situations. What started as an offhand comment has become a go-to phrase. Why is it in the language section? Because I have noticed that teachers and clinicians can talk a lot about too many things. B.K.S. Iyengar taught that yoga needs to be experienced. So trust the yoga experience. You do not have to state how a pose should feel and explain every last benefit. You also do not have to micromanage how someone does a pose. Teaching in a trauma-informed way builds body awareness because it gives someone the time and mental space to explore "what feels comfortable for you today." We will circle back to how your verbal pacing can support this teaching intention.

It is helpful to remember that you do not know how someone feels. You do not have all the answers. Pat Ogden, PhD, and Janina Fisher, PhD, remind us of the importance of adapting treatment to the needs of the individual rather than trying to fit someone into a treatment.[9] The psychologist Abraham Maslow, PhD, who developed the hierarchy of needs theory, is credited with saying that if all you have is a hammer, everything looks like a nail. You may want to consider how these ideas apply as you share trauma-informed yoga.

Keep It Literal and Body-Based: If your teaching intention is to build body awareness, then choose words that support building body awareness. I am not suggesting that more flowery, poetic language is wrong; such language can be quite beautiful. But I am suggesting that it could be distracting and confusing, and therefore not trauma-informed. Flowery language could be one more thing for a tired or stressed person to mentally process. How does a soft green light melting over sore muscles feel? "Notice if the stretch changes as you move from side to side" seems easier to follow. "Move your powerful breath to any tight areas in your back" seems vague when compared to the more specific "If you like, move until you feel a stretch across your shoulders." Literal and body-based language helps build body awareness with specific and clear cues. It can also help someone feel grounded by noticing what bodily sensations they are *feeling* now.

Limited Edition: While you may be excited to share what you know, keep in mind that more information is just that—more information to be processed. Time and energy to process your words is time and energy taken away from noticing how a breath feels today or finding a better way to move. Where appropriate, one cue and/or one benefit per pose can be enough to get someone set up and inspired. More information can be available as handouts (www.greentreeyoga.org/pain-management-resources).

Establish Boundaries for Time Keeping: We know that for someone who has experienced trauma, time can be an issue. Interestingly, the time-keeping part of the brain can go offline. People often feel stuck, a feeling that is also common to those in pain. A yoga practice teaching grounding techniques, linking the body and the breath, can help reactivate this part of the brain and regain a sense of time.[10,11] Again, it is body physiology.

So what cues support that this is now? Here are some ideas. "Always move in a way that is comfortable for you *today*." That one word, today, draws attention to time—simple to process, and simple for you to add. Another simple yet strong timekeeper is noting how many times you are going to practice something. For example, "We can practice 5 breaths." Or "The suggestion is to hold this stretch for 2 breaths. Hold the stretch…but not the breath." A clear number creates a boundary, allowing someone to physically experience that time passes. They are not stuck. But there is more.

Opportunity Knocks: Consider the empowering messages (yes, there is more than one) in: "The suggestion is to practice this flow 4 times. You can put your foot down any time; you are never stuck." What implied messages of opportunity does this cue hold for you? I found several. Opportunities to move within the safety of a time boundary: there is an end point. Opportunities for making small choices: "Do I want to practice this four times? Do I want to put my foot down?" Opportunities to practice flowing with breath and movement: "As YOU breathe in, arms lift... As YOU breathe out, arms release." Opportunities to gauge personal growth: "Last time I did two, but today it felt comfortable doing four." Opportunities to build a sense of curiosity: "I wonder if tree pose will feel different on this side today." Note that these messages are implied, meaning, I didn't say them out loud. Imagine if I had opened with "Okay, now here are some ways you can practice making small choices, get grounded in the present, feel the flow as we create connections between breath and movement, gauge your personal growth, oh, and maybe feel curious." Huh? A trauma-informed teaching idea is Show, Don't Tell. This simple approach can soothe a tired brain and body. (See Tables 5.1 and 5.2 for more ideas on phrases that support this approach.)

Let's pause for a moment to consider building a sense of curiosity. It is an important piece in trauma recovery, as noted by Bessel van der Kolk in his foundational and best-selling book, *The Body Keeps the Score*.[12] Supporting that idea, Bessel van der Kolk also explains that two of the most important phrases in trauma recovery are "notice that" and "what happens next."[13] His ideas are a natural fit for a trauma-informed yoga practice.

Absolutely Don't Do This: Why is it not responsible to speak in absolutes? Let's look at some examples. "A long breath out *will* lower blood pressure" or "A long breath in *will* energize you." For some, either breath can be agitating. Avoid the absolute with: "A long breath out *can* lower blood pressure." "Stretching your lower back muscles *will* decrease back pain" can become "Stretching lower back muscles *can* help to decrease back pain." Be aware that avoiding absolutes is teaching responsibly because it avoids telling someone what should happen. It will also build a sense of curiosity. Wait, what? Okay, it *may* build a sense of curiosity. Someone may notice if the stretch has an effect today. And that would be body awareness happening. Someone also won't feel like a failure if the stretch does not help today. Absolutely don't do this...

Use Consistent and Predictable Phrases: I was inspired to find phrases to use consistently after reading *My Voice Will Go With You*, a book by the eminent psychiatrist and hypnotherapist, Milton H. Erickson, MD.[14] He believed that everyone had within themselves all the tools they needed to heal, and that the role of the therapist was to help a person access those inner resources. One day a veteran said to me, "At home I heard your sweet little voice saying, 'Gently press one shoulder back, then press the other shoulder back.' My mother used to say 'stand up straight' not nearly as nicely." Someone chimed in that she heard the same thing at home. If you consistently use the same phrases, a few things can happen. Someone may hear your voice later, when they are at home or at work, and may need a bit of familiar and safe guidance. I have also had people say to me, "Well, you said, 'find a better way to move.' So, I tried." Or "Well, you said, 'always move in a way that is comfortable to me.'" I found it of interest that "well, you said" always started the comment. And to continue the point, here are two comments from refugee women in my community leader training: "I remember what you say, 'find a better way to move,' at night when I have pain in my legs." "I was just moving my shoulders and moving around... I heard you say, 'move when you can, stretch, don't be still.'" It wasn't exactly what I had said, but close enough. Consistent phrasing is also predictable. Therefore, it takes less mental energy to process. Aha, you may be thinking, someone will have more time and mental space to notice and become curious about what they are experiencing.

Use Some Repetition: I experienced the calming of simple repetition in a workshop with David Emerson. I still remember how it made me feel. He would give a simple cue. Then he would pause and simply repeat the cue in the same way. I remember *feeling* "Oh, okay, I have this..." It gave me a moment to find what he was suggesting without the distraction of new information. One way I have incorporated the idea is to say, "When you are ready, put one hand or both hands over your heart...put one hand or both hands over your heart." People tell me they like the rhythm of repetition.

Be Aware of Pacing: Let's pause for a moment to consider the pause. You may be from a region that tends toward speaking quickly or using a slower cadence. You may speak very quickly when you are nervous. Or you may feel long pauses make everything more yogic. As noted, someone needs time to process what we say. Then they need time to move slowly so they can "find a better way to move." There is a third piece to this sequence. Someone also needs time to notice their feelings and sensations after "moving and breathing in a comfortable way today." These three components create trauma-informed pacing: time to process, time to move, and time to notice. A well-timed pause gives someone those key moments in their practice. But the thread of your voice has not been lost.

Keep Talking—Your Voice Is a Thread to Safety: Why is it so important to keep talking? Stephen Porges explains in his books on polyvagal theory that a key gauge of safety for mammals comes from looking at faces and listening to voices.[15,16] Perhaps close your eyes now and imagine someone is talking. Can you tell if they feel safe or if they feel threatened? Now imagine they are speaking in a language you do not know. With your eyes closed and without understanding the words, do those vocal cues give information about the level of safety or danger in that room? And there you have it: your voice is a thread to safety.

Consider the social value of small talk. You may make eye contact with someone to add to the vocal exchanges that can cue levels of safety: "Haven't seen a storm like this in 20 years." To stay with the point, consider how you might feel if a stranger approaches you, head down, hands in pockets. Now consider how that feeling might change if, as they approach, they look at you, smile, and say, "Looks like Spring finally came."

Okay, but I did just suggest that you not share too many new ideas, and that you not distract with, well, too many words. So how does one stay true to your voice is a thread to safety without creating distractions? How does one not leave dead air, which could cause someone to wonder what they are supposed to be doing now or if something is wrong? Dead air can also cause someone to get stuck in the past because your voice is no longer there as a link, in real-time, to the present. So again, how do you keep that important thread?

> **The Takeaway: Perhaps give yourself a moment to look back at the previous few pages. Some suggestions on keeping the thread without being distracting include:**
>
> - Repeating the invitational phrases that resonate with you
> - Staying with body-based and literal cues to provide a link in real-time to body sensations
> - Using consistent and predictable phrasing, including repetition. (See the suggested phrases listed in Tables 5.1 and 5.2.)
>
> Be confident that these ideas work. A veteran in my pain class told me, "I have a hard time with that other teacher. He just talks all the time. You don't." I thought to myself, "But I do talk all the time. Always." But the difference? I talk about what we are doing. The other yoga teacher was also a therapist, and I think forgot the trauma-informed suggestion "to stay in your lane." You may want to add an awareness of your words and your pacing to what you practice. Ideas are outlined in this chapter's last section, Ways for You to Practice Your Trauma-Informed Teaching.

The Room

As Stephen Porges explains, a key point is that if someone does not feel safe, their energy and attention will go toward a defensive or a shutdown response.[17] It is body physiology. Therefore, promoting feelings of safety greatly improves any trauma recovery and pain management efforts. As Bessel van der Kolk reminds us, helping someone to learn self-regulation skills so they feel safe in their bodies is guiding a first step to trauma recovery. He says, "Emotional regulation is the critical issue in trauma."[18] So what can we do with the physical space to support this intention? There may be factors beyond your control. Outside noise, dirty carpets, crowded spaces, or flickering lighting come to my mind. Should you cancel the program? If there are no other location options, do not be discouraged.

The Art of Normalizing: A helpful rule of thumb is to control what you can and normalize what you cannot. Normalizing means to acknowledge that something is not unusual or abnormal. I taught a veterans' pain management class in a room that provided a wonderful opportunity to practice this approach. The room had a dirty carpet, every wall lined with workout equipment and things being stored, two years of construction noises outside the window, and courtesy carts in the hall, and well, you get the idea. However, I controlled what I could. I asked them to clean the carpet, which to my eye happened once a year. So I bought clean mats and clean cotton blankets. I brought in two floor lamps so I could turn off the flickering overhead lights. I always had a seasonal centerpiece in the middle of our circle, both to draw our circle together and to provide a focal point beyond the dirty carpet. I also always brought in baked goods to share after the class, which I thought added a positive safety cue, as well as sprigs of fresh herbs or evergreens to share.

How to Normalize: What I could not control, I normalized. I would say, "Looks like the guys are working on the prosthetics wing today, so expect noises." Or "The courtesy cart beeps when it backs up, so that will probably happen. It's a helpful service so folks don't have to walk in the long tunnel." Or "There are a lot of things in this room, but we still have all the room we need to practice today." I could easily have said, because it was true, "I have tried to get a better room, but they just keep telling me no. So, we are stuck here. I don't know why they can't store this stuff in the gym." With a bit of thought, you can let someone know that all is well, and you can, in fact, still practice. And you can add a bit of cheer wherever you can (clean mats, soft blankets, centerpieces, herbs).

Smelly Science: An interesting bit of science is that the strongest memory encoder is smell. For those interested, the signals go directly from the thalamus to the amygdala for an immediate reaction, no routing to the prefrontal cortex for thinking about it. It is the only sense that works in this way. Someone may not even know why a smell evokes a certain reaction. Note to your trauma-informed self: carefully consider what smells you introduce in the space. Lilacs tend to have a cloying smell. Incense and essential oils are designed to waft around a room. While well-intended, using strong scents takes away someone's option to choose. You are, in fact, introducing smells with potential triggers. I offer small sprigs of fresh herbs as they can help someone connect to the present situation, while the smells do not migrate to the next mat. Again, the response to a smell can be immediate and below the conscious radar. The physical response can also last long after the trauma that encoded it, which is one example of trauma being stored in the body. These ideas are good examples of what trauma-informed means. You are informed about some general trauma considerations.

Noisy Science: Low, deep tones can signal danger. As noted, if you expect such noises, simply say at the beginning of class, "The rumbling heat may come on with a loud clanging any time today." Now let's move to sounds you can control. Some teachers play music; some do not. The key is to do it with awareness, not as a reflexive action because it's what you think you should do. These classes are not your typical classes. Some teachers do not play music, preferring instead to create an environment with less external stimulation. Be aware that music with words can be distracting and even triggering. Banging drums can be…banging drums. The suggestion is, if you decide that gentle background music with no words is a good fit, keep it the same low volume the entire class. Being predictable and consistent are key trauma-informed gauges. If you have a sound system with issues, turn the music off. Irritation is not a good look on someone teaching self-regulation skills.

More Noisy Science: Breathwork can be a strong key to pain management. It's body physiology. But all breaths are not the same. As with anything you introduce into your trauma-informed space, be informed. Some breaths can be highly agitating—for example, those that cause sudden shifts in affect states (such as Tummo or Wim Hof breathing). Some breaths are just plain loud. Someone huffing or panting next to you, as in bellows breathing or Ouija breathing, can be less than ideal. Okay, they can be quite disturbing and triggering. One of the main takeaways for me from James Nestor's engaging book *Breath: The New Science of a Lost Art* (2020) is that breathwork is a powerful tool in affect regulation. His engaging melding of personal experiences, science, and cultural history is inspiring. But, like any tool, breathwork can be used and misused. Be mindful of what noises you introduce, and that includes breathing. Again (and again), be informed.

Light Up My World: Light is another sensory input, so how you work with lighting is important. Flickering fluorescent lights can be agitating. Based on your resources and your judgment, work with what you have. Bring in your own lighting if that is reasonable. Keeping the lighting consistent throughout the class can avoid sudden sensory shifts. If your room has windows and you know it will be getting dark, turning lights on at the beginning can keep the change more gradual. Turning the lights off near the end of a practice is another abrupt change to avoid. Again, work with what you have, but keep it consistent and minimize agitating shifts in sensory input, including sounds, lighting, and temperature.

How to Set Up the Room: Deciding how to use the available space is deciding how to build a sense of safety. A few trauma-informed considerations can guide you. Can someone easily see everyone in the room? Many feel more comfortable (safer) when no one is behind them or when their backs are not toward a door. The suggestion is to set up in a circle or semi-circle. Does someone have personal space defined by either a mat or a chair? If someone likes to be in the same spot every class, do you support that by saving their spot? Are there extra mats or chairs set up in your circle at the start of class so that if someone joins us later, no one has to experience the disruption of people and things moving? Can you teach in a small room with a big table in the middle or in a hospital room? Absolutely. You can share yoga in just about any situation, using safety and simplicity as a guide.

Props: In a trauma-informed class, the suggestion is to keep it simple. The only props I use are mats, chairs, and soft cotton blankets. Straps can be triggers for obvious reasons. I do not use yoga blocks, again, to keep it simple. In my experience, a chair and the floor can provide all the support needed. And if you are trying to plant some seeds of easy things to practice at home or at work, a chair can be the prop of choice. It is a great visual cue for practicing throughout the day: "Oh, a chair. I have two minutes to practice a stretch right here in my office (or kitchen)." I have also found that a chair can provide another safety cue. "Oh, I know this, how hard could it be?" Too many or unfamiliar props can create distractions and discomfort from the unknown. Again, the trauma-informed suggestion is to choose your props with awareness. You know your group.

Classroom Management

Isn't classroom management for schools? Well, yes. But let's learn a lesson as the same principles apply. You are creating a space in which to learn. In a trauma-informed class, you want to maintain a sense of safety so someone can learn new ways of managing stress and pain. You are teaching, but just as importantly, you are also managing. This idea may be a major shift for you. You may be used to arriving with your only responsibility being to teach. But again, this class is not your usual class. Some simple guidelines can help you to embrace your important role as a classroom manager.

Predictable and Consistent: Have the room set up before class starts, with the same props (chair, mat, blanket) for each class. Your presence is part of setting up the room. As everyone arrives, it is important that you are not attending to some administrative task somewhere else. Your presence in the room, again, is an important part of being predictable and consistent. It prevents the distraction of: "Is our teacher here today? What do I do now? Should I stay?" Again, you need to be part of the setup.

Welcome: Someone is "not late; they may be joining us later." Again, a few simple words can provide a positive spin. If you have set up a few extra spaces, someone joining you later can join seamlessly. They will not feel compelled to apologize or to explain, itself an interruption to your flow. "Welcome. Always move in a way that is comfortable for you today" relays that simple welcome. Someone hasn't interrupted. Your classroom is a predictable and welcoming place.

Safety: Let's pause to consider: "Always move in a way that is comfortable for you today." This simple cue does so much. Of course, the obvious—it empowers someone to be curious about what that comfortable way might be. It identifies that this is today, not yesterday. It also implies that you are not in charge of someone; they are. It implies you won't be watching them, looking for things to correct. Because part of classroom management is not asking about someone's issues, the cue prevents over-sharing. You have managed in a way to avoid triggering others. That one simple statement covers it.

And More Safety: Part of embracing your role as classroom manager is knowing how you want to address people who are, well, disruptive. And in a trauma-informed class, there is a broader definition of disruptive. Remember, your role is to build a feeling of safety for everyone. Be consistent in your responses. If someone is over-sharing with a list of what ails them or what happened to someone else, you can simply say, "The key to a good practice is to always move in a way that feels comfortable for you today. We can certainly chat after class." If people chatting is distracting, you can say, "Let's focus on our practice now. We can chat after class." You are clear, consistent, and, again, firm. This approach adds to the feeling of safety for everyone.

More About Disruptions: Again, there are things you can control and things you cannot. You can respectfully ask people to silence their phones during class. "Give yourself this time to focus on taking care of you, so let's all check and make sure our phones are silenced" can be effective. Something else you can and should control: staff, interns, or others who happen to join. You can be respectful, polite, and, again, firm. Embrace your role as someone who is managing the space. What does this mean? Imagine you have been invited to teach in a facility (school, treatment center, or community space). The staff may not know much beyond yoga seems like a good idea. It is not uncommon for staff to sit in the back chatting. Often they think they are being quiet, or they just haven't thought. You simply say, "You are welcome to join our practice, we have spots set up. But if you need to chat, would you please go out in the hall?" It is your space in which to do your job, whether paid or volunteer. If you are being paid, you should deliver the best product you can. If you are volunteering, you should deliver the best product you can. It's good to mention they are welcome to join us before class starts, but sometimes staff wander in. Again, control what you can in a respectful and firm way. Everyone will benefit.

All About You: Teacher, Clinician, or Healthcare Provider

Pieces of the puzzle that make up a trauma-informed room are the physical room and the participants. Again, you are also part of this physical space. That's right, whether a teacher, clinician, or healthcare provider—you are a part of the room. Let's consider how you can build safety, support empowerment, and maintain simplicity.

Your Fashion Statement: You may or may not put time into choosing what you wear. Consider that revealing yoga clothes, often both fun and appropriate in a fitness center, may be triggering or distracting in a trauma-informed setting. You may want to find clothing that is modest but that also allows people to see what you are suggesting. I used to wear scarves because I was cold, but people told me they couldn't see what I was doing. "Gently press one shoulder back, then press the other shoulder back" or "Notice if you have a gentle bend in your knees" are cues to model as you teach. Many of us benefit from visual cues. What you wear matters.

Hear All About It! Again (and again), be consistent and predictable in phrases and cues you bring into the room. It gives the verbal part of the brain less work to do, allowing someone to focus on how the movement or breath feels. Key phrases to support the intentions of safety, empowerment, and simplicity are listed in Tables 5.1 and 5.2. Examples of the many implied meanings in simple phrases are found throughout this book. Words matter.

Don't Hear All About It! I mention this because people have shared their feelings of discomfort and even dismay when teachers arrive and begin unloading their personal stressors. Consider how these actual comments set the emotional stage for a class. A teacher is late and spends the opening minutes explaining the woes of coordinating childcare with their ex-husband. A teacher is late and explains how they had to race down the freeway to get to class. A teacher is upset about another family issue...and well, you get the idea. A yoga class does not need to hear all about it. It can be triggering, and it is not appropriate in any class setting. The suggestion is to make leaving your personal concerns at the door part of your personal practice. The class can become a step-away respite for you.

Don't Phone It In: Polyvagal theory states that in addition to verbal cues, we gauge safety by reading facial expressions. It is not a small point. The foundational work of Paul Ekman, PhD, showed how across cultures people find the same feelings expressed in a smile or a face contorted in anger.[19] These studies support there being a biological, not cultural, basis for reading facial expressions. Based on this science, I offer three reasons to teach the poses and breathwork—not only stand there and talk. One is that many of us are visual learners, so looking at what you are suggesting can simplify the verbal cues. Another is that if you are just talking, some may feel you are watching them in search of things to correct. Most of us don't like to be watched. A third reason is that as you practice, it also affects your nervous system. You become a visual model for the flow of the calming or energizing effects of the poses and breathwork. That said, some attend my classes by phone, and it works well. But if you are in the room, take advantage of all teaching opportunities.

Be Relevant: No, this doesn't mean wearing the latest style or discussing the latest trends in goat yoga. It means keep your teaching relevant to someone's practice. It doesn't matter what you like, so saying "I really like this stretch" or "This breath really calms me down" is not relevant. The idea of relevance was brought home to me by a professor dealing with a lot of pain. As I started explaining the importance of a psoas stretch, she interrupted me with a laughing question, "Is this relevant to my practice?" I realized she was mentally fatigued as well and wanted simple suggestions with no added information. Be relevant...to someone's practice.

Do What You Say: If you tell someone you will bring something next week, make sure you do. You may be thinking, how important can that be? Offering something to look forward to provides two things that are important in trauma recovery, as Bessel van der Kolk explains. It helps build a sense of curiosity and a sense of time.[20] One older male veteran told me he looked forward to what flowers I was going to bring the next week, noting that I should have been a florist. I would tell people what the baked goods would be: "Next week I am baking blueberry cake, made from my sister's organic blueberries." You may have noted that it also builds social connections. Do what you say.

How You Keep Time: Another way to be consistent relates to time. If class starts at 1:00 pm, have the room set up on time. If there is another room activity that ends at 1:00 pm, identify your options. You may ask if that class could end at 12:55 pm. If that is not possible, as you all wait by the door, you can say, "Well, we will be able to get ourselves set up in a minute and get right to our practice." You are consistently okay with what happens, which models being flexible. Imagine the unease that could be caused if the room was not ready on time, and you were not there to model an adaptive response.

Your Many Messages: Let's circle back to the importance of vocal cues. Your voice and how you use it are what you bring into the room. Consider your response to a high-pitched, fast-paced string of words. What if the same words were said in a smooth, slow, gentle tone? While I am not suggesting that you take voice lessons, you may have more control over how you sound than you know. If you like, try this variation on imagining a voice. This time imagine someone calling your name from another room. How much information does that *one* word give you? Can you tell if someone feels afraid, angry, excited, or even tired? How can you tell? You only had the tone and cadence of their voice.

Be Nice to You: The idea bears repeating: be nice to you. In reviewing a class you've taught, you may notice you used some phrases you didn't mean to, that you forgot some aspect of setting up the room you had intended, or that something else didn't go as you had planned. The suggestion is to give yourself a lot of credit for noticing. Yes, noticing is important. Then you can decide what to do next time. The second suggestion is to be confident teaching with some trauma-informed protocols to build a sense of safety.

So, whatever didn't go quite right was experienced in this safer place. Daniel Siegel, MD, uses the term "widening the window of tolerance" to describe what might have happened.[21] You may have created a situation in which someone was able to increase their stress tolerance. So, be nice to you. Again, you noticed, and you can make adjustments.

> **A Quick Takeaway:** Set yourself up for success and spend some time on the last section of this chapter, Ways for You to Practice Your Trauma-Informed Teaching. You can start small, keep it simple, and build your program at your own pace. Becoming a trauma-informed teacher is a process.

Assists

This section is short and simple. In a trauma-informed class, the teacher does not move around the room. If you need to leave your spot to open the door or to bring someone an extra blanket, explain why you are moving and keep talking the whole time, ending with "I am now back on my mat." It may sound silly, but building a predictable and consistent sense of safety in the room is not silly.

Safety: Imagine a class in which the teacher suggests closing the eyes, at which point they quietly walk around the room putting their hands on people and telling them, "Do this, not that," and, well, you get the idea. Well-intended assists can be a distraction. "Is she coming over here? What will she do?" A teacher moving around could shift someone's awareness from "finding a comfortable way to move today" to wondering, "Am I doing this right? Will he think I am doing it wrong and come over to fix me?" In addition, you may not know someone's physical or emotional considerations. And remember, someone may not be aware of their triggers. Putting your hands on someone's hips may be a very strong trigger. Even lightly touching their arm may elicit a strong startle response. It is body physiology (hypervigilance). In addition, adjusting someone's shoulder based on how it looks is not helping to build body awareness, which comes largely from noticing how something feels. Instead, it may build self-consciousness as the focus shifts away from self to others.

Ways to Adjust: So how do we provide adjustments and still build a sense of safety? I have found two ways to be trauma-informed. One way is to use your words. Describe what you are suggesting. This approach supports noticing how a stretch or the breath feels today as opposed to how it looks to everyone else. You are helping someone to be present by "finding a better way to move," again, not a better way to look. Another way is to demonstrate with yourself as the visual cue: "It may be more comfortable to put your hand above your knee today."

All Together Now: Front and center in your trauma-informed teaching mind is that you do not want to single anyone out. Someone who has experienced trauma may not want to be called out for having made a mistake. One older veteran with a lifetime of trauma and pain texted me, "I try to be as inconspicuous as possible." Someone in pain may not want attention drawn to what they aren't able to do. And really, not many of us would appreciate such attention. An easy workaround is to offer adjustments to the entire group. "James, don't let your knee collapse in" can become "Okay everyone, if you like, tap your front leg. Now you can see my knee moving more toward center to protect my knee joint."

Not Part of the Plan: We know that human touch can be a powerful healing tool. But touch should be used in a proper therapeutic setting, one in which the teacher or healthcare provider has assessed each individual's need, and the necessary degree of trust has been established. Be informed: touch is not appropriate in a trauma-informed yoga group.

Teach to Empower

Empowerment sounds like an idea worthy of grand gestures. But to practice feeling empowered, small and simple gestures are a grand place to begin. Guide someone in simple breathing practices. Movements that stretch and strengthen can be gentle, even subtle, and the choices about how to practice them can be small. The steps are simple. Begin by guiding someone to notice where they are feeling the stretch or muscles working. If they notice and choose to make an adjustment, you have taught in a way that empowers.

Let's consider how mindful breathing, simple stretching, gentle strengthening, variations, and knowledge can create a wonderful synergy for empowerment.

Mindful Breathing

The science of breathing, complete with a short exercise to experience how breathing affects your nervous system in real-time, is discussed in Chapter 3. I used to teach breathwork as I had been taught, the teacher cueing when to breathe in, when to breathe out, and if and when to pause and for how long. You do what you know, as they say. But when a second veteran asked me in an agitated tone if he was breathing right, I realized I had failed. Rather than building an awareness of his personal breathing pattern, he was externally focused on me and on trying "to get it right." I spent some time thinking about how I could empower someone to feel confident managing their breathing. "Breathe in for the count of 6, then pause for the count of 6, then breathe out for the count of 6…" became "As YOU breathe in… As YOU breathe out." But the emphasis on *you* was not enough. If being trauma-informed is a body-based approach, not pairing more of the body with the breathwork seems a missed opportunity. In addition to stressing YOU, I link a body-based movement with the breath. Consider the empowering and grounding opportunities in: "As YOU breathe in, press down on your *fingertips*… As YOU breathe out, release the press." (See www.greentreeyoga.org/pain-management-resources for many other examples for you to practice and then teach, all linking self-directed breathwork with a simple or subtle movement.)

Don't Bury the Lede: If another breath experience would add a positive note to your day, here are two cues to do as you read them. "As you are ready, lift your arms toward the ceiling and take a breath in. Then, release your arms and breathe out." Next cue: "As YOU breathe in, lift your arms toward the ceiling… As YOU breathe out, arms release." Notice if the cues *felt* the same. Did one have a feeling of flowing? Did one feel choppier or disconnected? Of course, the answer is how it *felt* to you. Many have shared they felt a real difference. The second cue felt like a flow and much smoother. Perhaps try it one more time. The suggestion is don't bury the lede (the lead story in a news report), which is the breath in any yoga practice. Cue the breath first.

A Matched Set: I am often asked how you can match your breathing to those you are teaching. The answer becomes clear if you first consider your intention. Do you want to guide someone in practicing and choosing how to use their breath whenever they need it, day or night? Or do you want to tell someone what to do? If you try to match your breath to their breath, what are you teaching them? And do you want to match a breathing pattern that is choppy, shallow, or irregular? The suggestion is not to try. It may make you sound nervous as you realize you can't possibly match everyone. Empower someone to find and to practice a breathing pattern that serves their needs today. Instead of matching breaths, teach to empower, to notice, and to choose.

Simple Stretching and Gentle Strengthening

The phrase "simple stretching" has important considerations. Both the suggestions and the stretches should be simple to understand and simple to do. As mentioned before, someone in pain or in trauma recovery may have sleep challenges and be fatigued. Do you want their limited energy used to figure out what you mean or how to do a complicated stretch? Or do you want to set someone up for the success of experiencing the benefits of stretching: lowering muscle tension, reducing pressure on joints, reducing general stress levels, and decreasing some types of pain?

What makes a simple stretch should be determined by the person doing the stretch. I've had many people tell me the following cue was so helpful, but that it also took them a long time to give themselves permission to try it. "Small stretches, even a few centimeters or half an inch, can have benefits." Once someone stops trying to get somewhere with a stretch, something wonderful can happen. They can notice what "feels like a comfortable stretch today" and make adjustments as they go. They avoid the frustration and overstretching that can come with trying to do what a teacher tells them. Overstretching can also result in injury or in muscles being tighter than before the stretch. It's body physiology.

Another empowering idea is "Sometimes you do not know what stretch will feel comfortable until you try it, which is why the suggestion is to move slowly." One day my suggestion in Kitchen Stretch was "Move your hips until you find a comfortable stretch." One older woman with back pain, a clinical trauma diagnosis, and a great attitude said, "I know it's in here somewhere." Then, after a few breaths, she said, both surprised and pleased, "Oh, there it is!" Imagine if I had told her how she should move and then what it should feel like.

Teaching simple stretching should pose the same questions as teaching breathwork. Do you want to relay the message that "I know what is best for you, so do what I say?" Or do you want to empower someone to explore "finding new ways to move that feel comfortable for you today?"

Let's not forget these same considerations apply to gentle strengthening. In addition, someone noticing they feel stronger today and seeing personal growth can be empowering. Using the same trauma-informed protocols to teach strengthening poses also builds body awareness and is empowering. As the renowned author and teacher T.K.V. Desikachar notes, "Much more important than these outer manifestations is the way we *feel* the postures and the breath."[22]

Variations to Keep Everyone Engaged

Variations can empower as someone chooses when, or even if, to try something today. And if variety is the spice of life, then how can we follow the trauma-informed suggestion: "More is not better; more is confusing?" How do we keep it fresh without overwhelming or distracting someone with too much new information or too many choices? And how do we keep the flow of the practice while we spice it up?

A Firm Foundation of the Familiar: Let's first review why keeping some things the same is important in this program. As we discussed, consistent cueing is important because someone may hear your voice later. If someone wants to try Kitchen Stretch in their kitchen (or office), they can be guided by that solid base of the familiar. It also supports building a sense of safety through consistency and predictability. And as discussed, the familiar takes less energy to process, as someone already knows Tip-to-Toe Stretch or Finger Stretch Breath.

Spice It Up: If you are teaching the same group for many weeks, however, you can become so predictable that someone may stop listening. The trauma-informed suggestion is to change little things about the movement or your cueing, keeping the general pattern of the class consistent and predictable. For example, "When you are ready, stretch your arm to the side or toward the ceiling in a comfortable way. When you notice you are breathing…when you notice you are breathing, wiggle your fingers." The pose is the same, but you added a hand movement variation. Other small variations (only one at a time) are stretching the fingers wide, making a gentle fist, or pressing on the toes. Cueing in this way takes advantage of the high concentration of sensory receptors in both the hands and the feet. It also builds body awareness by creating a rhythm of breath and movement. The teaching intention is a little variety to keep someone (and yourself) mentally engaged, while again, empowering by choice. Many examples of variations are in the practice sequences in Part III.

Keep It Flowing: Another trauma-informed intention is to keep everyone engaged in the practice. If you stop to demonstrate all the variations, you have interrupted the practice flow. I have found two effective ways to keep it flowing. One way is: "Anything we do standing can be done seated or even lying down. You can always find ways to move and to breathe with me." I have observed people can find their own way, given your show of support offered by that simple cue. Again, be a guide and not a director.

Flowing in the Right Direction: Another way to teach variations is to present a flow with add-ons. Note that sequencing matters. If you like, do these stretches now. "As you are ready, stretch your arms toward the ceiling, fingers stretched wide. Or, if you want, you can stretch your arms to the side." Invitational language, literal language, so what's the problem? Now if you like, try it this way. "As you are ready, stretch your arms to the side, fingers stretched wide. Today you may want to stretch toward the ceiling. Different days, different stretches." You may have noticed in the first set of cues "your arms to the side" was added as something to do if you couldn't do what the teacher said. In the second cue "arms to the side" was the first suggestion, so someone might think, "I did it, success!" Anything more was simply something to try today. The order of the cues may seem like a small thing, but it isn't. Set someone up for success. Start with the gentler version, without using that word. Then you can offer, "Today you may want to do a *different* stretch." You can cue that different stretch, free of any judgment attached to such words as "stronger," "better," or "more advanced."

Knowledge Is Power
You may want to share helpful information. Consider, "You need to stretch your hamstrings because if you don't, tight hamstrings will add to back pain. Now step one foot forward…" Here is the same information in a different package: "Tight hamstrings *can* pull on your hip bone and may contribute to back pain. As you are ready, step one foot forward…" Notice the first example is directive, while the second cue is informational. Another example: "You need to take long, slow breaths out because it will calm you down. Breathe in…now take a long, slow breath out." Same information, different package: "Long, slow breaths out *can* lower heart rate and blood pressure. If you like, let's practice 5 breaths. As YOU breathe in, fingers press… As YOU breathe out, release." It is not a subtle difference. The first cue is directive with no choice. The second cue is informational, giving someone the option of using the information. If you want to teach to empower, present information that empowers someone to take charge of their day.

Let's consider one more example. A seemingly small change in the way you share information can provide a big opportunity to empower someone in their own pain management. You decide which cue empowers and which cue relays the message that someone isn't up to the task: "Building core muscles can help protect your back. You may want to begin with your hand on the chair and focus on the stretch. Or today you may want to take your hand off the chair to build core strength. Different days, different stretches. As you are ready…" Or "You need to build core muscles to help your back. Stand on one leg and balance for the count of 5. If you wobble, you can try again until you get it." Making what and how you share information a part of your teaching plan can greatly strengthen your teaching program. Again, another positive is that the process can keep you mentally engaged and interested, which is reflected in your voice.

Make a Plan

One day a woman said, "I did one of the breaths from last week at home. Was that okay?" I realized I had missed an important opportunity. I had not explained that what we practiced could easily be done at home or at work. As I thought about how to relay this information in a useful way, I came up with ending a practice with:

> If you would like, give yourself a moment to make a 2-minute plan to use later in the day or in the night when you would like to change how you are feeling. Perhaps pick one breath we practiced today—we did Finger Stretch Breath, feel the breath, and the Anytime, Anywhere Breath. Five long, slow breaths out *can* lower heart rate and blood pressure. Now, you might add 1 more minute to your break. If you like, choose one stretch we did today that you might want to do later. You now have a 2-minute plan to change how you are feeling.

After we have practiced making a plan in several classes, I might say: "Let's practice the breath you chose three times now. As YOU breathe in, hands move. As YOU breathe out, release." Cue the breath three times. After "Choose a stretch," I might say, "If you like, do that stretch now, so you have it ready to go."

These ideas are a strong start to Make a Plan, which you can then easily adjust to the needs of your group and yourself. Make a Plan is an important part of empowering someone to manage their pain. So, plan to have enough time at the end of your class, however long it is, to allow everyone to make their plan. It is also helpful to offer resources to take home, whether simple handouts, MP3s or MP4s (www.greentreeyoga.org/pain-management-resources).

Ways for You to Practice Your Trauma-Informed Teaching

You may be thinking that teaching in a trauma-informed way is a lot to think about. And you would be correct. But as in learning any new technique, having an easy plan can set you up for success. Let's consider your plan.

Make Your Plan: Again, shifting to a trauma-informed way of teaching is a process. The suggestion is to start small and, to stress the point, start small and set yourself up for success. Clipboard notes can be a strong starting point. All the sequences have clipboard notes to download, print, or edit to meet your needs (www.greentreeyoga.org/pain-management-resources). The two columns include the class outline, suggestions for time adjustments, and a place to write some key phrases you want to use. Before you dismiss using a clipboard by your mat or on your table as unprofessional, consider what it accomplishes. It shows you have taken the time to prepare, and you care about what you are sharing. You may sound more confident. Instead of using distracting filler words while you try to remember the next pose, your planned practice notes are right there. It also allows more of your attention to be on the participants. And again, the clipboard notes provide that base of the familiar to build a sense of safety and support empowerment. Consider that later someone may hear your voice in their mind, reminding them at home or at work of ways to lower stress. You can add or change phrases as feels comfortable to your teaching style. The suggestion is to use a clipboard proudly.

What You Say: The practice scripts were developed over many years of teaching workshops (www.greentreeyoga.org/pain-management-resources). Using feedback from participants who practiced with each other and later at home, I continued to change the scripts. What you find in this book reflects the combined contributions and observations of a diverse group of practitioners. The suggestion is to *first* practice the scripts as they are written. The real challenge, many have shared, is not to add words or little interesting things. Consider: More is not better; more is confusing. The scripts are based on trauma-informed ideas in this chapter. You can start teaching in a trauma-informed way with confidence. Then you can build your trauma-informed pain program to meet your personal and professional needs.

How You Sound: Ah, well, I sound like I sound, right? Until you give yourself a listen, you may not know how you sound, or even that you can change your sound. Here are some practice suggestions:

- **Record** (audio only) a few minutes as you read a stretching and breathing break from the practice scripts.
- **Listen** to the break as you do it along with your recorded voice. You may hear that you take long pauses as you teach, which is dead air. Or you may notice that your teaching voice is sing-song or monotone or too fast or that you sound nervous. You may want to re-record, using what you have learned. This exercise is a teaching tool for you. It can

be helpful to note pacing is the most commonly reported challenge. If you speak too quickly, someone may not have time to process, time to move, and time to notice. Again, if you leave dead air, you have missed an opportunity to use your voice as a thread to safety. You can develop the skills you need to teach in a way that finds a balance that supports your program.

- **Invite** someone to listen with you and as you do the break together. You can observe how that person responds and how it *feels* to you.

Supplemental Resources: Audio recordings (MP3s) of select practices are provided on the GreenTREE Yoga® website (www.greentreeyoga.org/pain-management-resources). Listening to the audio recordings may give you some ideas for your own classes. I would listen to a kids' yoga class as I drove to teach kids' classes, just to stay familiar with the tempo and the ideas in the class. I had written the script for the LittleTREE Yoga DVD, but I would hear Juliet's mellifluous voice in my head as I taught.

To Recap:

- The GreenTREE Yoga® Approach addresses trauma as it is held in the body. Peter Levine, PhD, who developed the Somatic Resourcing® program for body-based trauma recovery, reminds us that "trauma is primarily physiological."[23]
- How we use our language is a key to a trauma-informed approach. We can choose words that build a sense of safety, support empowerment, and maintain simplicity. Your voice can be a thread to safety, helping to anchor someone in the present.
- How you arrange the room directly affects the sense of safety in that space. You can make most spaces trauma-informed.
- To teach a trauma-informed class, you need to manage the group in a way that maintains a sense of safety for all.
- You are a part of the trauma-informed space. How you dress, what you do and say, and how you sound all affect that space.
- Using a trauma-informed approach may be new to you, or you may want to refine what you are already doing. There are some simple steps to support these efforts to set *you* up for success. Practicing the scripts can build your confidence as you build your program.

PART III

SIMPLE PRACTICES FOR EVERYONE

At Home, at Work, or in a Healthcare Setting

CHAPTER 5

Introducing the Sequences

This introduction serves as a quick review of key ideas discussed in previous chapters as well as a brief introduction for those who first want to explore the practice sequences. These practices support adaptability. Standing, seated, and lying down positions have different benefits. A variety of muscles are engaged and released as we arrange ourselves in different ways. The takeaway is that one position is not better than another.

For Personal Pain Management Strategies: You may be looking for simple pain management strategies to practice. You can be guided by following the practice sequences with photographs or by listening to select audio recordings. After experiencing the simple stretching, gentle strengthening, and mindful breathing, you may want to return to this introduction or to previous chapters for background information.

To Share Pain Management Strategies: If you are sharing this program with students, clients, or patients, these practice sequences, based on years of teaching and study, can be a strong start. This introduction supports my mantra: Be informed and be inspired.

Safety, Empowerment, and Simplicity: To recap, these pain management practices are designed to build safety, to support empowerment, and to maintain simplicity. These three ideas frame the GreenTREE Yoga® Approach. Building a personal sense of safety is key to pain management strategies. It decreases stress levels and creates a physiological condition (the biology of how living things function) for learning new things. Trauma-informed teaching empowers individuals to manage their nervous system and is part of every aspect of these practices. Regaining a sense of control can reduce stress. Information can also empower someone as they choose how to use that knowledge. Finally, maintaining simplicity is important because pain and trauma are often emotionally and physically exhausting. If your teaching style is simple to understand and simple to do, someone may have more mental and physical energy to notice how the movement and breathwork feel.

An Overview of Part III

Individual breathwork practices and poses are written according to the GreenTREE Yoga® Approach, used in all GreenTREE trainings, manuals, books, and audio/video recordings. The trauma-informed practice sequences in this book are written specifically for pain management. The short breaks and longer practice sequences include suggestions on how to create an effective practice. See Appendix A for the photographs.

Formats: The practices include: short breaks for work or home, 30-minute practices, and 60- to 90-minute practices. Practice sequences and select audio recordings (MP3s) and videos (MP4s) can support developing your personal or professional program. For example, someone could look at the practice sequences with the photos and perhaps listen to the audio recording. Then, simply listening to the audio recording to practice becomes an option. Again (and again), stretching and breathwork are about how it feels, not about how it looks. The audio recordings also offer teaching ideas on pacing and voice intonations that support healthy breathwork, gentle stretching, and strengthening techniques. Another practical option is to play the audio recording as you do the practice with a client, patient, or student.

Descriptions and Outlines: To help you choose a practice to meet your current personal and professional needs, this chapter includes short descriptions followed by the outline of each sequence.

Variations: Some practice sequences include variations. Offering one variation after someone is familiar with a pose or breathwork avoids distractions from information overload. A variation can keep interest and be empowering as someone notices personal growth. One variation may be offered for a specific breathwork or pose. A theme variation is included at the end of each practice to use after you have done the practice a few times. Variations can keep everyone engaged, including you.

Time Adjustments: Running out of time? Too much extra time? It's okay, you can make it part of your teaching plan. Here is another reason a list on your clipboard can be handy. Each practice sequence is designed to fill the allotted time, but teaching is, of course, more of an art than an exact science. To support your efforts to keep the flow, each sequence ends with time suggestions that honor the intention of that practice:

- **Running Out of Time:** Rather than abruptly stopping your flow or not leaving enough time for the all-important Make a Plan, specific ideas are outlined. Make a Plan is not an add-on if you have time; it is a key tool for empowerment. In the 60- to 90-minute practices, Final Stretch is not an add-on to be done if you have time; it is a key part of any longer practice, giving someone the time to reset the nervous system. I once heard it described as the time to "let the clay harden."

- **Too Much Extra Time:** Rather than winging it with poses that might not fit the flow, the suggestion is to say, "Let's now repeat some poses." The suggestions are listed. You have told people what to expect, so it will be a calming review of the familiar.

Trauma-Informed Language

The importance of language, both *what* you say and *how* you say it, is key to teaching trauma-informed yoga, as discussed in Chapter 4. To get a sense of the feelings that words can evoke, perhaps give yourself a few moments to read Tables 5.1 and 5.2. Notice how the phrases make you feel. Yes, notice how the phrases make you *feel*.

Table 5.1. Choices to empower

• Always move in a way that is comfortable for you today.	• Use the pieces of the stretch that feel comfortable for you today.
• If you want to change how you are feeling, perhaps breathe in a different way.	• Take your time with the stretch.
	• Find your own rhythm as you move and breathe.
• Always breathe in a comfortable way.	• You can make these stretches as gentle or as intense as you need today.
• Different day, different stretches.	
• You can always find ways to move and to breathe with me.	• You can change how you are stretching any time; you are never stuck.
	• The suggestion is to...

Table 5.2. Information to empower

• A long, slow breath out *can* lower blood pressure, lower heart rate, and lower muscle tension.	• Keeping your shoulders gently pressed back can reduce back strain.
	• When we do not move, tight muscles can press on nerves and joints.
• Moving even half an inch or a few centimeters has benefit. It means muscles are not getting tighter.	• As Moshé Feldenkrais said, "There isn't a right way to move; there is a better way to move."
• Visualizing a movement can have benefit.	• We move slowly so you can "find a better way to move."
• Anything we do standing can be done seated or lying down.	• We always do both sides.
• What is important is that it feels like a comfortable stretch for you today.	• A longer breath in *can* be energizing.

The phrases are intended to be nondirective, invitational, informative, simple, and empowering. Why are these phrases in easy-to-use tables? Repeating these simple phrases can build a sense of safety and support empowerment in every practice. A clinician told me that the language in my class was kind, which made my week. The suggestion is to teach using several phrases you choose and to notice the response.

Clipboard Notes: Whew, that is a long list of phrases. Set yourself up for success. As discussed in Ways for You to Practice Your Trauma-Informed Teaching in Chapter 4, using a clipboard allows you to be more confident in your teaching. If you have outlined your ideas, your teaching can stay simple, allowing you to teach to empower. (See www.greentreeyoga.org/pain-management-resources for clipboard notes for each sequence, which can be downloaded and edited.)

Seven Teaching Points

My pain management class took shape as I taught using these seven points. I wrote them down when I realized they reinforced simple ideas I wanted to share:

1. Managing YOUR breath:
   a. You can interrupt your stress cycle by choosing how you breathe.
   b. One way you can manage pain in real-time is by choosing how you breathe.
   c. Noticing your breath can be the first step in managing how you breathe.
2. Gentle stretching can reduce physical and emotional pain.
3. Moving slowly allows you "to find a better way to move."
4. Being aware of how you are sitting or standing (that is, your alignment) can help you manage pain.
5. Strengthening core muscles can reduce pain.
6. You can reduce pain or tension by not holding your breath.
7. Make a plan.

Information overload is not helpful in teaching, which is why these points are short and sweet. In the practice sequences, the opening cue is based on one or more variations of these seven points. It serves as a short and sweet reminder of why this practice is helpful in developing pain management strategies. Again, it uses repetition to support learning and to maintain simplicity. Be confident that these gentle reminders are helpful. I have been told by many, "Oh, I knew that, but I'd forgotten." Or "I really didn't know that, but it helps to understand why gentle stretching is helpful." Some simple information about the benefits of the practice can increase its effectiveness.

Let's take a few moments and consider how using these as opening cues can build safety, support empowerment, and maintain simplicity. Please note that the following explanations are only to inform how you teach and practice; they are *not* to explain during class, which truly would be information overload. Use the trauma-informed guide: More is not better; more is confusing. Participants often, however, appreciate handouts (www.greentreeyoga.org/pain-management-resources).

1. **Managing YOUR breath:**

    a. You can interrupt your stress cycle by choosing how you breathe.

    b. One way you can manage pain in real-time is by choosing how you breathe.

    c. Noticing your breath can be the first step in managing how you breathe.

    Each cue teaches a benefit of breathwork, which can be new information. A clear explanation is given in Chapter 3. The section on stress and the HPA axis might inspire you to take more care, both in how *you* breathe and how you teach breathwork. Using your breath to manage your stress cycle is an empowering piece of any pain management strategy. A focus of these practices is breath awareness, so it is heartening when someone says "I didn't know I was holding my breath until you said that thing…"

2. **Gentle stretching can reduce physical and emotional pain.** Many are grateful to have emotional pain acknowledged. Trauma and pain share neuronal pathways, so emotional pain is a real thing (the overlap is discussed in Chapter 3). All to say, a simple mention of emotional pain or tension can be validating. The information that even gentle stretching is helpful is also empowering.

3. **Moving slowly allows you "to find a better way to move."** Many of us are taught that working and pushing harder brings success.

It takes some gentle coaching to get comfortable with the idea that the practice is not to make your body do a specific movement or breath; the practice is "to find a way to move and to breathe that is comfortable for you today."

4. **Being aware of how you are sitting or standing (that is, your alignment) can help you manage pain.** The idea that how you sit or stand can affect pain is often new information. Healing from an injury or adjusting to pain can result in favoring one side. You may know other examples of how someone compensates for pain or injury. Some results include loss of strength on one side, tight muscles pulling on joints, or bones pressing on nerve roots. The practice sequences are designed to both increase awareness of and to improve posture and movement.

5. **Strengthening core muscles can reduce pain.** The idea that core muscles are important is familiar to many, but why that is true may not be. (See Strengthening: Alignment and Core in Chapter 2.) The short answer is that because core muscles wrap around you, front to back, they literally support good spinal alignment. Core muscles affect how your arms and legs function. Strengthening the core is not just about how it looks; strengthening the core is about how it feels. As you build core strength, do you hold yourself in better alignment, not leaning or favoring one side over the other? As you strengthen the core and stand in better alignment, do you notice less pain from muscles pulling on joints or bones pressing on nerve roots?

6. **You can reduce pain or tension by not holding your breath.** Typically, when we feel pain or discomfort, the first response is to brace and hold the breath. To use this approach over time is to create a stress response that may increase pain. The advice to just breathe through it is based in science. But it can be irritating when the advice doesn't offer a specific action to do in real-time. You may see where this is going. In Core Practice (II. Stretch, Breathe, and Strengthen Core), breathwork is practiced while strengthening the core. The Core Check practice is a continual favorite, which initially surprised me. Then I realized it builds both body awareness and empowers someone as they see personal growth from week to week. The Noticing Breath is a similar idea: noticing an area of emotional or physical discomfort and then taking long breaths out to lower heart rate and blood pressure.

7. **Make a Plan.** End strongly by empowering someone to make their one- to two-minute plan to use later as part of their pain management strategy. Just as breathwork is not an add-on to be done if you have time, making a plan is also not an add-on. Someone said to me, "I did that breathing at home, was that okay?" This comment taught me the importance of planting a seed and empowering someone with a plan to take home or to work.

A Closer Look: Practice Sequence Descriptions

Individual breathwork practices and poses are written according to the GreenTREE Yoga® Approach, used in all GreenTREE trainings, manuals, books, and audio/video recordings. The practice sequences in this book are designed specifically for pain management and building resiliency skills. The short breaks and practice sequences include suggestions on how to create an effective practice. See Appendix A for the photographs.

These yoga breaks and practice sequences can be used for many physical and emotional considerations. Choose a practice that meets the needs of most participants. Then you can support them in adapting their poses. This general outline of suggestions is a guide and not medical advice. Should you have any questions, please be evaluated by your healthcare provider to determine if simple stretching, gentle strengthening, and breathing exercises are a good choice for you or for your group(s).

Chapter 6: One- to Five-Minute Breaks: These short yoga breaks can be used at home, at work, or during a professional session. The suggestion is simple: use as needed. This chapter provides scripts and support materials for all the breathwork practices in this book, as well as ideas for pairing them with short movement practices.

Chapter 7: Thirty-Minute Practices: To create a strong base of the familiar, many of these poses and breathwork are found again, with variations, in the 60- to 90-minute flows in Chapter 8. Changing the sequencing creates different effects on both mind and body. It is...body physiology.

I. Stretch, Breathe, and Restore (Standing/Seated): Beginning with some large body movements linked to breathwork can decrease emotional and physical tension. Kitchen Stretch is introduced, using the familiar object of a chair to support stretching back and leg muscles. It also plants a seed to try this at home or at work. The sequence ends by finding a comfortable seat, to focus on shoulder, neck, and back stretches all linked to breathing.

II. Stretch, Breathe, and Strengthen Core (Standing/Seated): To reduce overall tension, the sequence starts with standing in the Tip-to-Toe Stretch. The option of using a chair, a safe and familiar prop, supports building core and exploring new stretching and strengthening options. "Different days, different stretches" is practiced here. Core Check practices breath awareness with a strengthening exercise.

III. Gently Moving Toward a Healthier Spine (Standing/Seated): This sequence includes ways to move toward a healthier spine: Tip-to-Toe Stretches; forward and back (flex and extend); side-to-side (lateral) stretches; and twists. All movements are done standing and then seated. This sequence provides the base of the familiar as it is expanded in Chapter 8 into a 60- to 90-minute practice to include lying down.

IV. Stretch and Breathe (Seated): Seated, either on the floor or in a chair, may provide the support someone needs to practice simple stretching, gentle strengthening, and mindful breathing. There are many ways to stretch from tip-to-toe from the safety of a seat.

V. New Ways to Stretch and Breathe (Kneeling/Seated): For someone wanting to stretch in new ways or for someone with an injury, kneeling with the arms on a chair seat offers a different approach to full body stretching. This variation of Kitchen Stretch gently stretches many muscles that may have tightened with extended sitting. Gentle movements and breathwork can be done from many body positions.

VI. Supported Stretch and Restore (Lying Down/Seated): Lying on a floor (or bed) allows some major muscle groups, which usually work to hold us upright, to release. Feeling the support of the floor can allow someone to focus more on the breathwork and stretching. Ending in a seated position allows for more focused shoulder and neck stretches. It can also provide a smooth transition to the rest of the day.

VII. Rest and Restore 1 (Lying Down): Some days 30 minutes of lying down has the most benefit. This sequence celebrates that even small stretches have benefits and visualizing a stretch has benefits. It allows someone to practice breathwork and moving in a gentle and supported way. This sequence has been called Jammie yoga, successfully done on a bed when someone is feeling fatigued.

VIII. Rest and Restore 2 (Standing/Seated/Lying Down): This sequence uses select standing and seated stretches with breathwork to prepare for the 15-minute Final Stretch, a body-based, guided meditation ending each

60- to 90-minute practice. It introduces an easy-to-use, easy-to-remember sequence to get to sleep or reduce stress. The trauma-informed meditation uses gentle tense-and-release cues guided by breathwork and the continual thread of your voice.

Chapter 8: Sixty- to Ninety-Minute Practices: Each practice uses physical flows connecting breath and movement to support the specific intention of the practice. Most of the poses and breathwork are found in the 30-minute practices, creating that strong base of the familiar. Some poses are new, and each sequence ends with the Final Stretch, a 10-minute, body-based, guided meditation. The strong suggestion is to leave a full 15 minutes for the Final Stretch, which includes Get Yourself Set Up; Final Stretch body-based, guided meditation (10 minutes); and Make a Plan to close.

I. Building Strength (Standing/Seated/Lying Down): Gently strengthening muscles and building flexibility can help manage pain. Standing stretches from tip-to-toe are complemented by strengthening exercises. Seated poses again include both strengthening and stretching, all linked to breathwork. The sequence concludes with lying down, continuing with the theme of stretching and strengthening.

II. Stretch, Breath, Rest, and Restore (Standing/Seated/Lying Down): Please note that this sequence is not a typical restorative practice with extended periods of quiet and stillness. It begins with some standing tip-to-toe stretches to release physical and emotional tension. Most of the postures are done lying down, but continued verbal guidance is provided. Again (and again), using your voice as a thread to safety combined with continual gentle movements and breathwork create this restorative practice.

III. Gently Moving Toward a Healthier Spine (Standing/Seated/Lying Down): This sequence expands the 30-minute practice of moving toward a healthier spine: tip-to-toe lengthening stretches; forward and back (flex and extend); side-to side (lateral) stretches; and twists. The fun part is moving each way in standing, seating, and lying down positions. The message is that you can move toward spinal health by moving and breathing in many supported ways.

In Case You Missed It...

These ideas are a quick reminder of why some words or phrases are used in these practice sequences. Each contributes to the important trauma-informed intention of building safety, supporting empowerment, and maintaining simplicity. Charlotte Bell's insightful and informative book, *Mindful Yoga, Mindful Life*, offers some guidance to anyone seeking to create a mindful yoga practice: "Mindfulness is the key to finding your own authentic yoga practice... When I am mindful, I can easily let go of ideas about yoga that do not fit, making room for new ways of seeing and practicing."[1] The following words and phrases support such a mindful practice, one that is empowering and that sets you up for success. So, in case you missed it...

1. **Tip-to-Toe or Raising Your Heart.** Why name everything? Naming provides an important reference so someone can know what you are about to do and can remember it later. "Oh, I know this, I like the Neck and Shoulder Suite we do at the end."

2. **"Gently press down on your toes..." or "Press on your fingertips..."** Why do so many cues involve fingers and toes? There are high concentrations of sensory receptors in the fingers and toes. Moving or pressing fingers or toes builds body awareness and is grounding, without any wordy or distracting explanations.

3. **"As YOU breathe in..."** Why stress YOU? Guiding breathwork, not dictating and micromanaging, can empower someone to notice and then to use their breath as a tool for pain management. Breathwork is a major pain management tool. Therefore, how you teach someone to manage their breath is critical to your program.

4. **"The suggestion is to practice this flow 4 times" or "Let's practice 3 breaths."** Why say the number of times? It provides predictability and allows someone to decide what they want to do today. It can also be a way for someone to gauge personal growth.

5. (*Say 3 times slowly*.) Speaking of numbers, why after "Let's practice 3 breaths" is "(*Say 3 times slowly*)" written? Some teachers would leave quiet after that cue. But it's trauma-informed to be a breathwork guide and not leave "dead air." Cueing each part of a breath is using your voice as a thread to safety.

6. **"The suggestion is..."** Using the word *suggestion* is a subtle way to remind someone you are not there to direct. And note that the suggestion is to use *the* suggestion, not *my* suggestion. Again, this is a subtle way to show you are guiding, not asserting control. Find every opportunity to be trauma-informed.

7. **"Gently press one shoulder back..." and "Gently move the fingers on one hand..."** Why start and end every breathwork practice the

same way? Gently moving the shoulders back physically sets someone up to take deeper breaths as they choose. It also gives a verbal and physical signal that breathwork is about to happen—it's an important thing to practice. Ending with moving the fingers or hands is another way to practice grounding and brings consistency to the important breathwork practice.

8. **"If you like, put one or both hands over your heart... Put one or both hands over your heart."** Why repeat the phrases? Simple repetition does three key trauma-informed things. It allows someone the time to decide what they want to do, to find a comfortable way in which to do it, and then to notice how it feels. It also keeps the thread of your voice going without adding distracting information to be processed by someone who may be fatigued.

9. **"...move in a way that is comfortable for you today."** Why is the word *today* used often? That one word can strengthen someone's connection to the present. This stretch may feel different today. Today it may be more comfortable to sit. Noticing that it is *today* can build body awareness and ground in the present.

10. **"Putting your foot on your knee can put extra pressure on that joint."** Why not say, "Don't put your foot on your knee?" Giving one simple fact can empower someone to decide how to use that information.

11. **Variations** can keep the practice interesting. Yet, to avoid too much information or too many choices, only offer one variation at a time after someone is familiar with that practice.

12. **"We move slowly to practice 'finding a better way to move' as we sit."** Why include "as we sit" or "as we lie down" in the opening cues? These simple phrases serve as a gentle reminder that we can stretch, strengthen, and breathe while standing, being seated, or lying down. Plant some seeds.

13. **"We always do both sides."** No, this cue is not a "duh" moment. If you say "right" or "left," it can be a distraction. Some will spend time and energy trying to do it correctly. This time and energy could be used to notice the stretch or the breath. Adopt the trauma-informed guide: "Simple to understand, simple to do." In a few flows, a right or left is needed as your point of reference, but the cue still includes "We always do both sides."

14. **"You are never stuck."** Someone in chronic pain may feel stuck. The simple statement can be a gentle reminder that they have choices. Many have told me how they like that phrase.

15. **"There isn't a right way to move; there is a better way to move."** Reminding someone that you have no expectations and that small stretches have benefits takes just that: reminding someone. It's a shift from typical class expectations of getting it right by doing what the teacher says.

16. **"Let's practice this 3 times" or "We practice slowly so that…"** Why is the word *practice* used so much? That simple word sends a message of support. We are all always practicing; there is no end goal or point we need to reach. To my mind, practicing meets someone where they are.

CHAPTER 6

One- to Five-Minute Breaks

Introduction

Support for You: You may be looking for short, simple breaks for your own pain management plan to use at home or at work. Or you may want to use some breaks in your professional setting. Either way, this chapter provides easy-to-use resources. Scripts, handouts, MP3s (audio), and MP4s (video) provide support (www.greentreeyoga.org/pain-management-resources). The breathwork and simple stretching breaks are from the longer practice sequences in Chapters 7 and 8. Repetition is a way to become familiar with and gain confidence in using the breaks. The suggestions work in a wide variety of settings and provide a strong starting point. As you develop your program to do at home or at work, you can add favorites from the following chapters.

Timing Is Everything: Starting a session by lowering stress levels and creating grounding opportunities can help you or someone with whom you are working create a more receptive physiological state. Or, more simply, a short breathing or stretching break can turn it around. The same benefits apply when using a break mid-session as a step-away. Lastly, a break to close a session can provide a positive ending note by grounding with self-regulation skills and body awareness. One breathwork practice or one simple stretch, as outlined in Tables 6.1 and 6.2, creates a one- to two-minute break. Pairing a breathwork practice with a simple stretch creates a longer break, as outlined in Table 6.3. The breaks work well together, so mix and match as meets your interest and pain management needs.

Setup for Success: Practicing also sets the stage for Make a Plan. It is empowering to practice a break and then have the handout, the MP3, or MP4 to use later. Setting up for success can be as easy as playing the audio recording of the break and doing the break with a client, student, or patient. It's a break for you, too.

Keep It Simple: The suggestion is to keep it simple, offering or learning one break at a time. In keeping with the trauma-informed idea of simplicity, the suggestion is to share resources for one break at a time. And in the spirit of not overwhelming someone (or yourself), please note that the variations are to try after someone is familiar with the breaks.

These breaks are not medical advice. Please consult your healthcare provider if you have any questions about the benefits of simple stretching and mindful breathing for you or for those with whom you work.

Table 6.1. Single breathing breaks (see www.greentreeyoga.org/pain-management-resources for handouts, MP3s, and MP4s)

Breathing 1: Feel the Breath (2:10)
Breathing 2: Choose your breathing pattern (2:23)
Breathing 3: Fingertip Press (2:20)
Breathing 4: The Wave Breath (2:11)
Breathing 5: The Physiological Sigh (2:16)
Breathing 6: Anytime, Anywhere Breath (2:54)
Breathing 7: The Noticing Breath (2:30)
Breathing 8: Thumb to Fingertip Press (2:42)
Breathing 9: Finger Stretch Breath (2:21)
Bonus Breaths
Breathing Bonus 10: Choose your breath and Finger Stretch Breath (4:07)
Breathing Bonus 11: Get Unstuck: Feel the Breath, The Wave Breath, and Thumb to Fingertip Press (6:10)

Table 6.2. Single stretching breaks (see www.greentreeyoga.org/pain-management-resources for handouts, MP3s, and MP4s)

Stretching 1: Tip-to-Toe Stretch (2:14)
Stretching 2: Wide-Legged Add-On (2:08)
Stretching 3: Shoulder Rolls (2:35)
Stretching 4: 1-2-3 Shoulder Stretch (2:03)
Stretching 5: Shoulder Rock 'n Roll (3:08)
Stretching 6: Find a New Stretch (2:19)
Stretching 7: Seated Cat/Cow (2:25)

Table 6.3. Breathing and stretching short pain management breaks (see www.greentreeyoga.org/pain-management-resources for handouts, MP3s, and MP4s)

Break 1: Shoulder Rolls and Finger Stretch Breath (3:50)
Break 2: Tip-to-Toe Stretch, Shoulder Rolls, and Finger Stretch Breath (5:21)
Break 3: Physiological Sigh, Shoulder Rock 'n Roll, and Feel the Breath (5:20)
Break 4: 1-2-3 Shoulder Stretch, Find a New Stretch, and Finger Stretch Breath (5:24)
Break 5: Tip-to-Toe Stretch, Wide-Legged Add-On, and The Wave Breath (5:35)
Break 6: Wide-Legged Add-On and Feel the Breath (4:06)
Break 7: Seated Cat/Cow, Find a New Stretch, and Feel the Breath (5:47)
Break 8: Tree Pose and Choose Your Breath (3:16)
Break 9: Kitchen Stretch (6:58)
Break 10: Neck and Shoulder Suite (10:26)
Lying Down Breaks
Break 11: Hip-to-Toe Stretch (14:47)
Break 12A: Final Stretch (8:51)
Break 12B: Bonus Final Stretch (13:35)

Breathwork (photos on p.262)
Feel the Breath

Key Phrase: Long breaths out *can* lower heart rate, lower blood pressure, and lower muscle tension.

Opening Cue: One way we can manage pain in real-time is by choosing how we breathe.

Cues:

1. When you are ready, gently press one shoulder back... Then press the other shoulder back.
2. If you like, put one or both hands over your heart... Put one or both hands over your heart.
3. The suggestion is to practice 5 breaths. Feel the breath in... Feel the breath out.
   (*Say 2 times slowly.*) Always breathe in a comfortable way. Feel the breath in... Feel the breath out.
   (*Say 3 times slowly.*)
4. If you like, gently move the fingers on one hand or shake that hand... Then gently move the fingers on the other hand or shake that hand.

Feel the Breath with Fingertip Press

Key Phrases: (1) Longer breaths in *can* be energizing. (2) Long, slow breaths out *can* lower blood pressure. (*Or choose one of these phrases based on what fits the needs of the class.*)

Opening Cue: One way we can manage pain in real-time is by choosing how we breathe.

Cues:

1. When you are ready, gently press one shoulder back... Then press the other shoulder back. If you like, put one or both hands over your heart... Put one or both hands over your heart.
2. Let's practice 5 breaths. Feel the breath in, fingertips press... Feel the breath out, release the press. (*Say 2 times slowly.*)
Always breathe in a comfortable way.
Feel the breath in, fingertips press... Feel the breath out, release. (*Say 3 times slowly.*)
3. If you like, gently move the fingers on one hand or shake that hand... Then gently move the fingers on the other hand or shake that hand.

Finger Stretch Breath

Key Phrase: A long, slow breath out *can* lower heart rate, lower blood pressure, and lower muscle tension.

Opening Cue: Noticing your breath can be the first step in managing how you breathe.

Cues: In Finger Stretch Breath, the suggestion is to stretch your fingers half an inch or a few centimeters. (**Variations.**)

1. When you are ready, gently press one shoulder back... Then press the other shoulder back. If you like, let's practice 5 breaths.
2. As YOU breathe in, fingers stretch... As YOU breathe out, release. (*Say 2 times slowly.*) Always breathe in a comfortable way. On YOUR next breath in, fingers stretch... As YOU breathe out, release.
As YOU breathe in, fingers stretch... As YOU breathe out, release. (*Say 2 times slowly.*)
3. If you like, gently move the fingers on one hand or shake that hand... Then gently move the fingers on the other hand or shake that hand.

Variations: (1) Stretch just enough to notice the stretch. **Or** (2) Stretch your fingers as wide as you would like today. **Or** (3) Perhaps stretch your fingers in a different way today.

The Wave Breath

Key Phrase: Long, slow breaths out *can* lower heart rate, lower blood pressure, and lower muscle tension.

Opening Cue: Noticing your breath can be the first step in managing how you breathe.

Cues:

1. When you are ready, gently press one shoulder back... Then press the other shoulder back.
2. The suggestion is to take 5 breaths as we practice the Wave Breath.
   As YOU breathe in, hands lift (*palms up*)... As YOU breathe out, release (*palms down*). (*Say 2 times slowly.*)
   Always breathe in a comfortable way. On YOUR next breath in, hands lift... As YOU breathe out, release. As YOU breathe in, hands lift... As YOU breathe out, release. (*Say 2 times slowly.*)
3. If you like, gently move the fingers on one hand or shake that hand... Then gently move the fingers on the other hand or shake that hand.

Physiological Sigh

Key Phrase: Practicing the physiological sigh 2 or 3 times can help lower carbon dioxide levels in the blood, which can lower anxiety.

Opening Cue: You can interrupt your stress cycle by choosing how you breathe.

Cues:

1. When you are ready, gently press one shoulder back... Then press the other shoulder back.
   Let's practice once. Always move and breathe in a comfortable way. When you are ready, practice a deep breath in and stretch your fingers wide. Then breathe in more; perhaps stretch your fingers a little more. Hold that breath as long as you like...when you are ready, SIGH it out, fingers release. The suggestion is to practice 2 more times. (*Say 2 more times.*)
2. The physiological sigh is a way to practice lowering your anxiety levels in 2 or 3 breaths.
3. If you like, gently move the fingers on one hand or shake that hand... Then gently move the fingers on the other hand or shake that hand.

The Noticing Breath

Key Phrase: Long, slow breaths out *can* lower heart rate, lower blood pressure, and lower muscle tension.

Opening Cue: You can interrupt your stress cycle by choosing how you breathe.

Cues: Notice if you have any area in which you feel discomfort—either physical or emotional. Or pick an area on which to practice—your knee, perhaps.

1. The Noticing Breath is 5 breaths. The suggestion is long, slow breaths out, if that is comfortable for you today.
2. When you are ready, gently press one shoulder back... Then press the other shoulder back.
3. On YOUR breath in, notice that area of discomfort... On YOUR breath out, keep noticing. (*Say 2 times slowly.*) Instead of ignoring the discomfort, the suggestion is to keep noticing it as you breathe.
4. On YOUR next breath in, notice that area... On YOUR breath out, keep noticing.
   On YOUR breath in, notice that area... On YOUR breath out, keep noticing. (*Say 2 times slowly.*)
5. If you like, gently move the fingers on one hand or shake that hand. Then gently move the fingers on the other hand or shake that hand.
6. You may want to practice the Noticing Breath later, when you want to interrupt your stress cycle.

Anytime, Anywhere Breath

Key Phrase: Long, slow breaths out can lower heart rate, lower blood pressure, and lower muscle tension.

Opening Cue: One way we can manage pain in real-time is by choosing how we breathe.

Cues: You can do the Anytime, Anywhere Breath even when talking with someone.

1. When you are ready, gently press one shoulder back... Then press the other shoulder back. If you like, place one hand on your leg in a way that is comfortable for you today.
2. Let's practice 5 breaths. The suggestion is to take long, slow breaths out. (**Variation 1.**)

As YOU breathe in, fingers press... As YOU breathe out, release. (*Say 2 times slowly.*) Always breathe in a comfortable way.
On YOUR next breath in, fingers press... As YOU breathe out, release. As YOU breathe in, fingers press... As YOU breathe out, release. (*Say 2 times slowly.*)

3. If you like, gently move the fingers on one hand or shake that hand... Then gently move the fingers on the other hand or shake that hand. (**Variation 2.**)
4. You may want to practice the Anytime, Anywhere Breath later, when you want to change how you are feeling.

Variations: (1) Press your fingers firmly or gently today. **Or** (2) Now if you like, use your other hand and practice saying it 3 times to yourself in your mind, since *you* are always with you. (*Say slowly during this time so you don't leave "dead air:" Don't rush your words... Don't rush your breath. Take your time with your words... Take your time with your breath.*)

Simple Stretching
Tip-to-Toe Stretch (photos on p.243)

Key Phrase: Always move in a way that is comfortable for you today.

Opening Cue: One way to manage pain is with gentle stretches to reduce pressure on nerves and joints.

Cues:

1. When you are ready, stretch one arm to the side or overhead, fingers stretched wide in the Tip-to-Toe Stretch.
2. Then stretch the other arm, either to the side or overhead, fingers stretched wide.
3. Find your own rhythm as you stretch one arm and then the other. Take your time with each stretch. (**Variation.**)
4. When you are ready, put your hands on your hips.
If you like, lift one heel and press on your toes. Then lift the other heel and press on the toes. Let's practice that 2 more times. (*Say 2 times slowly.*)

Variation: Today you may like to arc one arm overhead and then the other. Find your own rhythm as you move.

Wide-Legged Add-On (photos on p.245)

Key Phrase: Moving even half an inch or a few centimeters has benefits; it means muscles are not getting tighter.

Opening Cue: As Moshé Feldenkrais said, "There isn't a right way to move; there is a better way to move."

Cues:

1. When you are ready, step your feet apart, hands on your hips as we do the wide-legged add-on. (**Variation.**)
2. In whatever way feels comfortable, move one hip to one side... Then move the other hip to the other side. We move slowly so you can "find a better way to move."
3. Today you may like to add lifting your shoulder in a gentle arc as you move to one side... Then lift the other shoulder in a gentle arc as you move the other hip to the side. Find your own rhythm as you move from side to side. Take your time as you move.
4. When you are ready, come back to standing tall. If you like, gently *stretch* the fingers on one hand or shake that hand... Then gently *stretch* the fingers or shake the other hand.

Variation: Today you may want to roll from the inside edges to the outside edges of your feet... Roll from the inside to the outside edges in any way that is comfortable for you today.

Shoulder Rolls (photos on p.254)

Key Phrase: Today you may want to practice long breaths out.

Opening Cue: Long breaths out *can* reduce muscle tension.

Cues:

1. If you like, let's practice 3 shoulder rolls forward and 3 shoulder rolls back. As YOU breathe in, shoulders lift... As YOU breathe out, shoulders roll forward and down. Always move in a comfortable way. (*Say 3 times slowly.*)
2. Now 3 back. As YOU breathe in, shoulders lift... As YOU breathe out, shoulders roll back and down. (*Say 3 times slowly.*)

Variations: (1) After one roll: if you like, move even more slowly on the next two rolls. **Or** (2) After two rolls: if you like, stop halfway down this last roll. Hold the stretch...but not your breath.

1-2-3 Shoulder Stretch (photos on p.254)

Key Phrases: (1) Even small stretches have benefits. (2) Long, slow breaths out *can* lower blood pressure.

Opening Cue: The suggestion is to practice 1-2-3 Shoulder Stretch 3 times.

Cues:

1. Gently bend your elbows if that is comfortable for you today.
2. As YOU breathe in, press both shoulders back… That's 1.
   As YOU breathe out, press both shoulders forward… That's 2.
   And release… That's 3. And that's 1 set. You can make each stretch as gentle or intense as you need today.
3. The suggestion is to practice 2 more sets of 1-2-3 Shoulder Stretch. (*Say slowly 2 more times.*)

Shoulder Rock 'n Roll (photo on p.254)

Key Phrase: Different days, different stretches.

Opening Cue: Moving slowly allows you "to find a better way to move" as we practice 3 sets of shoulder Rock 'n Roll.

Cues:

1. Gently bend your elbows and stretch your fingers if that is comfortable for you today.
2. When you are ready, move one arm across the front, the other arm across the back, as we practice shoulder Rock 'n Roll. Leading from the elbows if you like, now move the other arm across the front, and the other across the back. That's 1 set. Find your own rhythm as you practice 2 more sets. You can make each stretch as gentle or as intense as you need today. Moving the arms from front to back in any way that feels comfortable… Finding your own rhythm as you move.
3. Now if you like, lead from the shoulders as you move from front to back. Practice as many sets as feels comfortable for you today… Moving the arms from front to back as slowly as you would like.
4. Now, the suggestion is to hold the stretch on each side for 2 breaths. As one shoulder moves across the front and the other across the back, hold the stretch…but not your breath. Feel the breath in…feel the breath out. (*Say 2 times slowly.*)
5. Now as your other shoulder moves across the front and the other across the back, hold the stretch…but not your breath. Feel the breath in…feel the breath out. (*Say 2 times slowly.*)
6. When you are ready, arms to your sides.

Find a New Stretch
Cues:

1. Give yourself a few moments to create some simple stretches as you stand, sit, or lie down. You can move with me or find your own ways to stretch. (*Cue what you are doing as you move.*) Perhaps move your arms in a new way, one arm and then the other. Notice if you stretch your fingers wide. Then move both arms in a new way.
2. If you like, step your feet apart and move from side to side. Perhaps moving your hips in a circle is a new way to stretch today. Take your time as you move in a comfortable new way.
3. Now the suggestion is to take up space on the last stretch. If you like, put more effort into your breath in as you stretch your fingers and toes and arms. Take up space as you breathe and stretch in a comfortable way.
4. When you are ready, come back to standing or sitting tall.

Seated Cat/Cow (photos on p.242)
Key Phrase: Different days, different stretches.

Opening Cue: Let's continue to lengthen spinal muscles to create more space between the bones in the spine (vertebrae).

Cues:

1. If you like, tap your *fingertips* on your legs. The suggestion is to practice seated cat/cow 2 times.
2. As YOU breathe in, chin lifts...shoulders back...rock forward.
As YOU breathe out, chin tucks...shoulders forward...rock back a comfortable distance. Always move and breathe in a comfortable way. On YOUR next breath in, chin lifts...shoulders back...rock forward. As YOU breathe out, chin tucks...shoulders forward...rock back a comfortable distance.
3. When you are ready, come back to sitting tall.
4. If you like, let's practice 2 more breaths. As YOU breathe in, press down on all your fingers and all your toes. As YOU breathe out, release. (*Say 2 times slowly.*)

CHAPTER 7

Thirty-Minute Practices

Outlines and Practice Sequences

I. Stretch, Breathe, and Restore (Standing/Seated)
A. Standing

1. Tip-to-Toe Stretch
2. Wide-Legged Add-On
3. Feel the Breath
4. Kitchen Stretch: a. Setup; b. Strong and Steady; c. Hip Rock 'n Roll; d. Hamstrings and Calf Stretch; e. Wrap Up

B. Seated

1. Get Yourself Set Up
2. Finger Stretch Breath
3. Cat/Cow
4. Shoulder Suite: a. Lift and Release; b. Forward and Back; c. 1-2-3 Shoulder Stretch; d. Shoulder Rock 'n Roll; e. Find Your New Stretch
5. The Noticing Breath

C. Make a Plan

D. Extras

1. Time Adjustments
2. Theme Variation: Little Changes

II. Stretch, Breathe, and Strengthen Core (Standing/Seated)

A. Standing

1. Tip-to-Toe Stretch
2. Feel the Breath with Fingertip Press
3. Wide-Legged Add-On
4. Hip Stretch and Core Strengthening Flow: a. Pendulum and Pedal the Feet; b. Hip Spirals; c. Hip Circles; d. Feel the Breath; e. Warrior 3 Flow

B. Seated

1. Get Yourself Set Up
2. Core Check
3. Finger Stretch Breath
4. Fancy Footwork
5. Find Your New Stretch
6. Anytime, Anywhere Breath

C. Make a Plan

D. Extras

1. Time Adjustments
2. Theme Variation: The Pause

III. Gently Moving Toward a Healthier Spine (Standing/Seated)

A. Standing

1. Tip-to-Toe Stretch
2. Feel the Breath
3. Side-to-Side (Lateral) Stretches: a. Crescent Stretch; b. Wide-Legged Add-On
4. Cat/Cow (Flex and Extend)
5. Twist: Ring the Bell
6. Tip-to-Toe Stretch

B. Seated

1. Get Yourself Set Up
2. The Wave Breath
3. Tip-to-Toe Stretch
4. Side-to-Side (Lateral) Stretches: a. Shoulder Lift and Release; b. Crescent Stretch
5. Cat/Cow (Flex and Extend)
6. Twists: a. Shoulder Rock 'n Roll; b. Classic Twist with Cat/Cow
7. Anytime, Anywhere Breath

C. Make a Plan

D. Extras

1. Time Adjustments
2. Theme Variation: Savor the Stretch

IV. Stretch and Breathe (Seated)
A. Seated

1. Get Yourself Set Up
2. Tip-to-Toe Stretch
3. Feel the Breath
4. 1-2-3 Shoulder Stretch
5. #4 Stretch: a. #4 Flow; b. #4 Twist; c. Cat/Cow
6. Finger Stretch Breath
7. Eagle Flow: a. Eagle Wrap; b. Eagle Wrap in a Twist; c. Cat/Cow
8. Fancy Footwork
9. Quads and Psoas Stretch with Cat/Cow
10. Neck and Shoulder Suite: a. Neck Massage; b. Chin Lifts and Pendulum; c. Neck and Shoulder Stretches
11. Feel the Breath with Fingertip Press

B. Make a Plan

C. Extras

1. Time Adjustments
2. Theme Variation: Stretch the Toes

V. New Ways to Stretch and Breathe (Kneeling/Seated)
A. Kneel 'n Stretch

1. Get Yourself Set Up
2. Hip Rock 'n Roll
3. Feel the Breath with Fingertip Press
4. Psoas and Glutes Stretch
5. Wide Knee Stretches
6. Quads and Psoas Stretches/Twist
7. Hip Rock 'n Roll
8. Cat/Cow

B. Seated

1. Get Yourself Set Up
2. Tip-to-Toe Stretch
3. Physiological Sigh
4. Shoulder Rolls
5. Find a New Shoulder Stretch
6. Fancy Footwork
7. Neck and Shoulder Suite: a. Neck Massage; b. Chin Lifts and Pendulum; c. Neck and Shoulder Stretches
8. Feel the Breath

C. Make a Plan

D. Extras

1. Time Adjustments
2. Theme Variation: The Pause (Take 2)

VI. Supported Stretch and Restore (Lying Down/Seated)
A. Lying Down with Supported Spine

1. Get Yourself Set Up
2. Feel the Breath
3. 1-2-3 Shoulder Stretch
4. Gentle Twist with Knees

5. Bridge Flow: a. Raising Your Heart; b. Bridge Lift and Release; c. Side-to-Side Rocking

B. Seated

1. Get Yourself Set Up
2. Tip-to-Toe Stretch
3. Finger Stretch Breath
4. Neck and Shoulder Suite: a. Neck Massage; b. Chin Lifts and Pendulum; c. Neck and Shoulder Stretches
5. Shoulder Rock 'n Roll
6. Shoulder Rolls
7. Feel the Breath
8. Physiological Sigh

C. Make a Plan

D. Extras

1. Time Adjustments
2. Theme Variation: The Pause (Take 2)

VII. Rest and Restore 1 (Lying Down)
A. Lying Down

1. Get Yourself Set Up
2. Feel the Breath
3. Tip-to-Toe Stretch
4. Bridge Flow: a. Raising Your Heart; b. Bridge Lift and Release
5. Hip-to-Toe Stretches: a. Toes, Foot, and Ankle 1; b. Toes, Foot, and Ankle 2; c. Knee Stretch; d. Spiral Hip Stretch; e. Outer Hip Stretch/Twist; f. Back Release 1
6. Feel the Breath with Fingertip Press
7. 1-2-3 Shoulder Stretches: a. 1-2-3 Single Shoulder Stretch; b. 1-2-3 Double Shoulder Stretch; c. 1-2-3 Side-to-Side Shoulder Stretch
8. Back Release 2: Knee Circles
9. Tip-to-Toe Stretch
10. Anytime, Anywhere Breath

B. Make a Plan

C. Extras

1. Time Adjustments
2. Theme Variation: Savor the Stretch

VIII. Rest and Restore 2 (Standing/Seated/Lying Down)
A. Standing

1. Tip-to-Toe Stretch
2. Wide-Legged Add-On

B. Seated

1. Get Yourself Set Up
2. Feel the Breath
3. Cat/Cow
4. Shoulder Rolls

C. Lying Down

1. Get Yourself Set Up
2. Final Stretch: A Body-Based, Guided Meditation

D. Seated

1. Get Yourself Set Up
2. 1-2-3 Shoulder Stretch
3. Finger Stretch Breath

E. Make a Plan

F. Extras

1. Time Adjustments
2. Theme Variation: Savor the Stretch

PRACTICE SEQUENCES

I. STRETCH, BREATHE, AND RESTORE (STANDING/SEATED)

Note: Before you teach, please review In Case You Missed It... (p.101)

A. Standing
1. Tip-to-Toe Stretch (photos on p.243)

Key Phrase: Always move in a way that is comfortable for you today.

Opening Cue: One way to manage pain is with gentle stretches to reduce pressure on nerves and joints.

Cues:

1. When you are ready, stretch one arm to the side or overhead, fingers stretched wide in the Tip-to-Toe Stretch.
2. Then stretch the other arm, either to the side or overhead, fingers stretched wide.
3. Find your own rhythm as you stretch one arm and then the other. Take your time with each stretch. (**Variations.**)
4. When you are ready, put your hands on your hips.
   If you like, lift one heel and press on your toes. Then lift the other heel and press on the toes. Let's practice that 2 more times. (*Say 2 times slowly.*)

Variations: (1) Today you may like to arc one arm overhead and then the other. Find your own rhythm as you move. **Or** (2) As you stretch one arm, lift the heel on the other side. Find your own rhythm as you stretch the arm and lift the other heel. When you are ready, stretch one arm and lift the heel on the same side. Move in a comfortable way, stretching and lifting. Then if you like, keep practicing the way that was more of a challenge.

2. Wide-Legged Add-On (photos on p.245)

Key Phrase: Moving even half an inch or a few centimeters has benefits; it means muscles are not getting tighter.

Opening Cue: As Moshé Feldenkrais said, "There isn't a right way to move; there is a better way to move."

Cues:

1. When you are ready, step your feet apart, hands on your hips as we do the wide-legged add-on. (**Variation.**)
2. In whatever way feels comfortable, move one hip to one side... Then

move the other hip to the other side. We move slowly so you can "find a better way to move."
3. Today you may like to add lifting your shoulder in a gentle arc as you move to one side... Then lift the other shoulder in a gentle arc as you move the other hip to the side. Find your own rhythm as you move from side to side. Take your time as you move.
4. When you are ready, come back to standing tall. If you like, gently *stretch* the fingers on one hand or shake that hand... Then gently *stretch* the fingers or shake the other hand.

Variation: Today you may want to roll from the inside edges to the outside edges of your feet in a comfortable way... Roll from the inside to the outside edges in any way that is comfortable for you today.

3. Feel the Breath (photo on p.262)

Key Phrase: Long breaths out *can* lower heart rate, lower blood pressure, and lower muscle tension.

Opening Cue: One way we can manage pain in real-time is by choosing how we breathe.

Cues:

1. When you are ready, gently press one shoulder back... Then press the other shoulder back.
2. If you like, put one or both hands over your heart... Put one or both hands over your heart.
3. The suggestion is to practice 5 breaths. Today you may like to practice long breaths out.
   Feel the breath in... Feel the breath out. (*Say 2 times slowly.*) Always breathe in a comfortable way.
   Feel the breath in... Feel the breath out. (*Say 3 times slowly.*)
4. If you like, gently move the fingers on one hand or shake that hand... Then gently move the fingers on the other hand or shake that hand.

4. Kitchen Stretch (a/b/c/d/e) (photos on pp.249–250)
A. SETUP

Key Phrase: Even small stretches have benefits.

Opening Cue: Gently stretching muscles can move you toward a healthier spine.

Cues:

1. Let's practice 3 moves to protect your back and knees as you bend forward. Gently press your shoulders back, press your hips back a small amount, and keep a slight bend in your knees.
2. The suggestion is to interlace your fingers and rest your forearms on the back of the chair. If you draw your elbows in so they line up with your shoulders, you won't be hanging on your shoulder joints. (**Variation.**)
3. When you are ready, release forward a comfortable distance, as we practice Kitchen Stretch.

Variation: Today you may want to press your palms together. Perhaps try something different.

B. STRONG AND STEADY

Key Phrase: You can adjust your feet; you are never stuck.

Opening Cue: Gently stretching back and leg muscles can move you toward a healthier spine.

Cues: The suggestion is to take 4 breaths as we do strong and steady. You may want to practice long, slow breaths out today.

1. As YOU breathe in, feel the press on the chair... As YOU breathe out, press your hips back any distance. (*Say 4 times slowly.*) When you are ready, come back to standing tall.
2. If you like, practice 3 shoulder rolls back. As YOU breathe in, shoulders lift... As YOU breathe out, shoulders roll back and down. (*Say 3 times slowly.*)

C. HIP ROCK 'N ROLL

Key Phrase: You can make the stretches as gentle or intense as you need today.

Opening Cue: Gently lifting and tucking the tailbone can help keep spinal discs healthy.

Cues:

1. Stand tall with your hands on your hips. Give yourself a moment to tuck your tailbone. Then lift your tailbone. One more time...tuck your tailbone and then lift your tailbone. Notice you can do this motion without moving your legs. This lifting and tucking motion is hip Rock 'n Roll.

2. When you are ready, gently press your shoulders back, hips back, and slightly bend your knees. Then get yourself set up again for Kitchen Stretch.
3. Find your own rhythm. As YOU breathe in, lift your tailbone... As YOU breathe out, tuck your tailbone. Take your time as you lift and tuck in hip Rock 'n Roll several times. Always move and breathe in a comfortable way.
4. The suggestion is next time you lift your tailbone, hold the stretch for 2 breaths. Hold the stretch...but not your breath. Feel the breath in... Feel the breath out. (*Say 2 times slowly.*) Next time you tuck your tailbone, hold it for 2 breaths. Hold the stretch...but not your breath. Feel the breath in... Feel the breath out. (*Say 2 times slowly.*)

D. HAMSTRINGS AND CALF STRETCH (PHOTO ON P.250)

Key Phrase: Tight hamstrings can pull on the hip bone and cause back pain.

Opening Cue: We move slowly so you have time "to find a better way to move."

Cues:

1. When you are ready, adjust your Kitchen Stretch so it is comfortable for you today. Then step one foot back.
2. Notice you have a bend in your front knee as you gently press that hip back. Release forward a comfortable distance.
3. Perhaps massage the hamstring muscles, the top back part of your leg. Take your time with the stretch.
4. The suggestion is to practice 3 more breaths here. Feel the breath in... Feel the breath out. (*Say 3 times slowly.*)
5. When you are ready, come back to standing. Then get yourself set up with the other leg forward. (**Repeat.**)

E. WRAP UP

If you like, let's end by doing Strong and Steady again. (**Repeat b.**)

B. Seated
1. Get Yourself Set Up

Key Phrases: (1) Anything we do seated can be done standing or even lying down. (2) You can always find ways to move and to breathe with me.

Opening Cue: Sitting or standing with your shoulders gently pressed back can take pressure off your back.

Cues:

1. Give yourself a few moments to find a comfortable way to sit today, either on a folded blanket or on a chair.
2. Gently press one shoulder back... Then press the other shoulder back.
3. If you like, move from side to side as you settle into your seat. Perhaps move in a circle. Take your time as you move. You may want to circle even more slowly the other way.
4. Make any adjustments to find a more comfortable seat.

2. Finger Stretch Breath (photo on p.262)
Key Phrase: A long, slow breath out *can* lower heart rate, lower blood pressure, and lower muscle tension.

Opening Cue: Noticing your breath can be the first step in managing how you breathe.

Cues: In Finger Stretch Breath, the suggestion is to stretch your fingers half an inch or a few centimeters. (**Variations.**)

1. When you are ready, gently press one shoulder back... Then press the other shoulder back.
2. If you like, let's practice 5 breaths. As YOU breathe in, fingers stretch... As YOU breathe out, release. (*Say 2 times slowly.*)
   Always breathe in a comfortable way.
   On YOUR next breath in, fingers stretch... As YOU breathe out, release.
3. As YOU breathe in, fingers stretch... As YOU breathe out, release. (*Say 2 times slowly.*)
4. If you like, gently move the fingers on one hand or shake that hand... Then gently move the fingers on the other hand or shake that hand.

Variations: (1) Stretch just enough to notice the stretch. **Or** (2) Stretch your fingers as wide as you would like today. **Or** (3) Perhaps stretch your fingers in a different way today.

3. Cat/Cow (photos on p.242)
Key Phrase: Different days, different stretches.

Opening Cue: Let's continue to lengthen the spinal muscles to create more space between the bones in the spine (vertebrae).

Cues:

1. If you like, tap your *fingertips* on your legs. The suggestion is to practice seated cat/cow 2 times.
2. As YOU breathe in, chin lifts…shoulders back…rock forward.
   As YOU breathe out, chin tucks…shoulders forward…rock back a comfortable distance.
   Always move and breathe in a comfortable way.
3. On YOUR next breath in, chin lifts…shoulders back…rock forward. As YOU breathe out, chin tucks…shoulders forward…rock back a comfortable distance.
4. When you are ready, come back to sitting tall.
5. If you like, let's practice 2 more breaths. As YOU breathe in, press down on all your fingers and all your toes. As YOU breathe out, release. (*Say 2 times slowly.*)

4. Shoulder Suite (a/b/c/d/e) (photos on p.254)

A. LIFT AND RELEASE

Key Phrase: Even small stretches have benefits.

Opening Cues: Gentle stretching can reduce physical and emotional pain. Let's practice the Shoulder Suite.

Cues: The suggestion is to start with 3 sets of lift and release.

1. When you are ready, gently lift one shoulder…release the other shoulder. Then gently lift that shoulder…and release the other. That's 1 set.
2. Always move in a comfortable way as we do 2 more sets. (*Say 2 more times.*)

B. FORWARD AND BACK

Key Phrase: You can make these stretches as gentle or as intense as you need today.

Cues: Now let's move in a different way with 3 sets of forward and back.

1. When you are ready, arms by your sides as you press one shoulder forward…and press the other shoulder back. Then press that shoulder forward…and the other back. That's 1 set.
2. Find your own rhythm as we practice 2 more sets. (*Say 2 more times.*)

C. 1-2-3 SHOULDER STRETCH

Key Phrases: (1) Even small stretches have benefits. (2) Long, slow breaths out *can* lower blood pressure.

Opening Cue: The suggestion is to practice 1-2-3 Shoulder Stretch 3 times.

Cues:

1. Gently bend your elbows with fingers stretched wide if that is comfortable for you today.
2. As YOU breathe in, shoulders and elbows press back... That's 1.
As YOU breathe out, shoulders and elbows press forward... That's 2.
And release... That's 3. And that's 1 set. You can make each stretch as gentle or intense as you need today.
3. The suggestion is to practice 2 more sets of 1-2-3 Shoulder Stretch. (*Say slowly 2 more times.*)

D. SHOULDER ROCK 'N ROLL

Key Phrase: Different days, different stretches.

Opening Cue: Moving slowly allows you "to find a better way to move" as we practice 3 sets of shoulder Rock 'n Roll.

Cues:

1. Gently bend your elbows and stretch your fingers if that is comfortable for you today.
2. When you are ready, move one arm across the front, the other arm across the back as we practice shoulder Rock 'n Roll. Leading from the elbows, if you like, now move the other arm across the front, and the other across the back. That's 1 set. Find your own rhythm as you practice 2 more sets. You can make each stretch as gentle or intense as you need today. Moving the arms from front to back in any way that feels comfortable... Finding your own rhythm as you move.
3. Now if you like, lead from the shoulders as you move from front to back. Practice as many sets as feels comfortable for you today... Moving the arms from front to back as slowly as you would like.
4. Now, the suggestion is to hold the stretch on each side for 2 breaths. As one shoulder moves across the front and the other across the back, hold the stretch...but not your breath. Feel the breath in... Feel the breath out. (*Say 2 times slowly.*)
5. Now as your other shoulder moves across the front and the other across the back, hold the stretch...but not your breath. Feel the breath in... Feel the breath out. (*Say 2 times slowly.*)
6. When you are ready, arms to your sides.

E. FIND A NEW SHOULDER STRETCH

Key Phrase: Moving slowly allows you to practice 'finding a better way to move'.

Opening Cue: Gentle stretches can help reduce both physical and emotional pain.

Cues:

1. To finish the Shoulder Suite, give yourself a few moments to move your shoulders in a new way. If you like, you can follow me or find your own new stretches. (*Slowly cue the stretches you are doing.*)
2. Notice if you feel a new stretch today.
3. If you like, gently move the fingers on one hand or shake that hand... Then, gently move the fingers on one hand, or shake that hand.

5. The Noticing Breath

Key Phrase: Long, slow breaths out *can* lower heart rate, lower blood pressure, and lower muscle tension.

Opening Cue: You can interrupt your stress cycle by choosing how you breathe.

Cues: Notice if you have any area in which you feel discomfort—either physical or emotional. Or pick an area on which to practice—your knee, perhaps.

1. The Noticing Breath is 5 breaths. The suggestion is long, slow breaths out if that is comfortable for you today.
2. When you are ready, gently press one shoulder back... Then press the other shoulder back.
3. On YOUR breath in, notice that area of discomfort... On YOUR breath out, keep noticing. (*Say 2 times slowly.*) Instead of ignoring the discomfort, the suggestion is to keep noticing it as you breathe.
   On YOUR next breath in, notice that area... On YOUR breath out, keep noticing.
   On YOUR breath in, notice that area... On YOUR breath out, keep noticing. (*Say 2 times slowly.*)
4. If you like, gently move the fingers on one hand or shake that hand. Then gently move the fingers on the other hand or shake that hand.
5. You may want to practice the Noticing Breath later, when you want to interrupt your stress cycle.

C. Make a Plan

Opening Cue: Next time you start to feel pain or discomfort, you can have a 1- or 2-minute plan ready to go.

Cues:

1. The suggestion is to choose one breath we did today. We did Feel the Breath, Finger Stretch Breath, and the Noticing Breath. Long breaths out *can* lower blood pressure. So now you have a 1-minute breath to do later when you want to change how you are feeling.
2. If you like, add one stretch you might like to do again—maybe the wide-legged add-on or Kitchen Stretch. You now have a 2-minute plan to manage your pain.

(See www.greentreeyoga.org/pain-management-resources for free downloads.)

D. Extras
1. Time Adjustments

Running Out of Time? When you notice you are running out of time, move ahead to the Noticing Breath. Then Make a Plan.

Too Much Time? After the Noticing Breath, stand again and repeat the Tip-to-Toe Stretch, wide-legged add-on, and Finger Stretch Breath. Then find a comfortable seat to Make a Plan.

2. Theme Variation: Little Changes

After you have done this practice several times, you can offer this idea at the beginning and mention it a few times during the practice:

> Today, you might want to do the stretches in a different way. You can make little changes as we move and breathe.

II. STRETCH, BREATHE, AND STRENGTHEN CORE (STANDING/SEATED)

Note: Before you teach, please review In Case You Missed It... (p.101)

A. Standing
1. Tip-to-Toe Stretch (photos on p.243)

Key Phrase: When we do not move, tight muscles can press on nerves and joints.

Opening Cue: As Moshé Feldenkrais said, "There isn't a right way to move; there is a better way to move."

Cues:

1. When you are ready, stretch one arm to the side or overhead, fingers stretched wide in the Tip-to-Toe Stretch.
2. Then stretch the other arm, either to the side or overhead, fingers stretched wide.
3. Find your own rhythm as you stretch one arm and then the other. We move slowly so you can "find a better way to move." (**Variations.**)
4. When you are ready, put your hands on your hips. The suggestion is to lift one heel and press on your toes. Then lift the other heel and press on the toes. Let's pedal the feet two more times. (*Say 2 times slowly.*)

Variations: (1) Today you may like to arc one arm overhead and then the other. Find your own rhythm as you move. **Or** (2) As you stretch one arm, lift the heel on the other side. Find your own rhythm as you stretch the arm and lift the other heel. When you are ready, stretch one arm and lift the heel on the same side. Move in a comfortable way, stretching and lifting. Then if you like, practice the way that was more of a challenge.

2. Feel the Breath with Fingertip Press (photo on p.262)

Key Phrases: (1) Longer breaths in *can* be energizing. (2) Long, slow breaths out *can* lower blood pressure. (*Or choose one of these phrases based on what fits the needs of the class.*)

Opening Cue: One way we can manage pain in real-time is by choosing how we breathe.

Cues:

1. When you are ready, gently press one shoulder back... Then press the other shoulder back. If you like, put one or both hands over your heart... Put one or both hands over your heart.
2. Let's practice 5 breaths. Feel the breath in, fingertips press... Feel the breath out, release the press. (*Say 2 times slowly.*) Always breathe in a comfortable way.
   Feel the breath in, fingertips press... Feel the breath out, release. (*Say 3 times slowly.*)
3. If you like, gently move the fingers on one hand or shake that hand... Then gently move the fingers on the other hand or shake that hand.

3. Wide-Legged Add-On (photos on p.245)

Key Phrase: Moving even half an inch or a few centimeters has benefits; it means muscles are not getting tighter.

Opening Cue: Another way we can manage pain is with gentle stretches to reduce pressure on nerves and joints.

Cues:

1. When you are ready, step your feet apart, hands on your hips as we do the wide-legged add-on. (**Variation.**)
2. In whatever way feels comfortable, move one hip to one side… Then move the other hip to the other side. We move slowly so you can "find a better way to move."
3. Today you may like to add lifting your shoulder in a gentle arc as you move to one side… Then lift the other shoulder in a gentle arc as you move the other hip to the side. Find your own rhythm as you move from side to side. Take your time as you move.
4. When you are ready, come back to standing tall. If you like, gently *stretch* the fingers on one hand or shake that hand… Then gently *stretch* the fingers or shake the other hand.

Variation: Today you may want to roll from the inside edges to the outside edges of your feet in a comfortable way… Roll from the inside to the outside edges in any way that is comfortable for you today.

4. Hip Stretch and Core Strengthening Flow (a/b/c/d/e) (photos on p.253)

A. PENDULUM AND PEDAL THE FEET

Key Phrase: Different days, different stretches.

Opening Cue: Another way to manage pain is to strengthen muscles, especially the core muscles that wrap around the front and back and help keep your spine in alignment.

Cues: A slight bend in your standing leg will protect the knee joint.

1. We always do both sides. When you are ready, slowly move your leg from side to side, like a pendulum.
2. You may want to take your hand off the chair as you move. You build core strength as you move to find your balance. When your hand is on the chair, you can focus on the stretch.
3. When you are ready, put your foot down and your hands on your hips.

4. Give yourself a moment to lift one heel, press on the toes. Then lift the other heel, press on the toes. If you like, practice 2 more sets, making the press as firm or as gentle as you need today.

B. HIP SPIRALS

Key Phrase: Always move in a comfortable way.

Opening Cue: We can strengthen core muscles as we find our balance.

Cues:

1. When you are ready, move your leg in a circle, a spiral, or any comfortable way.
You may want to take your hand off the chair as you move. Again, you build core muscles as you find your balance. It's like lifting arm weights but using yourself.
2. Then, perhaps move even more slowly in the other direction. When you are ready, put your foot down.
3. Give yourself a moment to pedal your feet 3 times. Lift one heel…press on the toes. Lift the other heel…press on the toes. Today, you may like to add to the stretch: roll onto the tops of your toes and then roll over and press down. (*Say 3 times slowly.*)

C. HIP CIRCLES

Key Phrase: Take your time with the stretch.

Opening Cue: Let's continue to stretch muscles and lubricate the hip joint as we find our balance.

Cues:

1. When you are ready and still standing on the same leg, move your leg in a wide arc, as if your toe is drawing a circle front to back around the standing leg.
2. You may want to take your hand off the chair as you move. Then circle your foot in the other direction. When you are ready, stand tall.

D. FEEL THE BREATH

Key Phrase: Longer breaths in *can* be energizing.

Opening Cue: Noticing your breath can be the first step in managing how you breathe.

Cues:

1. When you are ready, gently press one shoulder back... Then press the other shoulder back.
2. If you like, put one or both hands over your heart... Put one or both hands over your heart.
3. The suggestion is to take 3 breaths. Feel the breath in... Feel the breath out. (*Say 3 times slowly.*)
4. If you like, gently move the fingers on one hand or shake that hand... Then gently move the fingers on the other hand or shake that hand.

E. WARRIOR 3 FLOW (PHOTOS ON P.253)
Key Phrase: Different days, different stretches.

Opening Cue: Tight hip and leg muscles can pull on your hip bone and cause back pain.

Cues:

1. (*Hand on or off the chair.*) When you are ready, lift your knee a comfortable distance to stretch the glutes.
2. Then stretch your leg toward the back to stretch the front hip flexor. Move the leg forward and back in a comfortable way.
3. When you are ready, hold one stretch, leg forward or back. Hold the stretch...but not your breath. When you notice you are breathing...when you notice you are breathing, wiggle your fingers.
4. When you are ready, put your foot down. Give yourself a moment to pedal your feet again, gently stretching the thick layers of muscles and connective tissue in your feet. Again, you may like to add to the stretch and roll over the toes and press down. (**Repeat a/b/c/d/e on the other side.**)

B. Seated
1. Get Yourself Set Up
Key Phrases: (1) Anything we do seated, you can do standing or even lying down. (2) You can always find ways to move and to breathe with me.

Opening Cue: Sitting or standing with your shoulders gently pressed back can take pressure off your back.

Cues:

1. Give yourself a few moments to find a comfortable way to sit today, either on a folded blanket or on a chair.

2. Gently press one shoulder back... Then press the other shoulder back.
3. If you like, move from side to side as you settle into your seat. Perhaps move in a circle. Take your time as you move. You may want to circle even more slowly the other way.
4. Make any adjustments to make your seat more comfortable.

2. Core Check (photos on pp.247–8)

Key Phrases: (1) Gently pressing your shoulders back can relieve back pain. (2) You always can change the way you are moving; you are never stuck.

Opening Cues: Practicing long breaths out when you feel discomfort can interrupt your stress cycle. Building core strength can protect the back. Let's practice both now as we do Core Check.

Cues:

1. When you are ready, sit forward on your chair or a folded blanket.
2. Gently press one shoulder back... Then press the other shoulder back.
3. Slide your hands back. If you feel any burning, numbness, or tingling, adjust your stretch.
4. Notice your next breath in... On YOUR breath out, release back until you feel some core muscles working. Moving even half an inch or a few centimeters has benefits.
5. Take 2 breaths here if you like. As YOU breathe in, fingers stretch... As YOU breathe out, release. (*Say 2 times slowly.*) When you are ready, come back to sitting tall. That was you building core muscles and not holding your breath. You might like to say quietly, "Check."
6. The suggestion is to do this gentle strengthening 4 more times. Notice that one shoulder is still back...and that the other shoulder is back. As YOU breathe in, hands press... As YOU breathe out, release back. Today perhaps lift one leg. (**Adapt variations for your group.**)
7. When you feel muscles working, take 2 more breaths. As YOU breathe in, fingers stretch... As YOU breathe out, release. (*Say 2 times slowly.*) Come back to sitting tall. "Check." You just practiced building core muscles and not holding your breath when feeling some discomfort. (*Say 3 more times slowly.*)

Variations: (1) Lift one or both arms to shoulder height as you release back. **Or** (2) Lift one leg (knee bent or leg straight) as you release back. **Or** (3) Lift both arms and one or both legs as you release back.

3. Finger Stretch Breath

Key Phrase: Long, slow breaths out *can* lower heart rate, lower blood pressure, and lower muscle tension.

Opening Cue: You can interrupt your stress cycle by choosing how you breathe.

Cues: In Finger Stretch Breath, the suggestion is to stretch your fingers half an inch or a few centimeters. (**Variations.**)

1. When you are ready, gently press one shoulder back… Then press the other shoulder back. If you like, let's practice 5 breaths.
2. As YOU breathe in, fingers stretch… As YOU breathe out, release. (*Say 2 times slowly.*) Always breathe in a comfortable way. On YOUR next breath in, fingers stretch… As YOU breathe out, release.
   As YOU breathe in, fingers stretch… As YOU breathe out, release. (*Say 2 times slowly.*)
3. If you like, gently move the fingers on one hand or shake that hand… Then gently move the fingers on the other hand or shake that hand.

Variations: (1) Stretch just enough to notice the stretch. **Or** (2) Stretch your fingers as wide as you would like today. **Or** (3) Perhaps stretch your fingers in a different way today.

4. Fancy Footwork (photos on pp.260–1)

Key Phrase: As Moshé Feldenkrais said, "There isn't a right way to move; there is a better way to move."

Opening Cue: Stretching the thick layers of muscles in the feet and ankles can ease pressure on joints and improve circulation.

Cues:

1. When you are ready, lift your leg a comfortable distance and put your hands around your shin or back of your leg.
2. Gently press one shoulder back… Then press the other shoulder back to take stress off your back.
3. If you like, slowly move this foot in a circle… Then circle the other way. (**Variation.**)
4. Give yourself a moment to move your foot in a new way, taking your time with the stretch.
5. If you like, stretch all your toes 3 times. As YOU breathe in, stretch your

toes... As YOU breathe out, release. (*Say 3 times slowly.*) (Repeat on the other side.)

Variation: When you are ready, move the foot 3 times from side to side, like a windshield wiper. Now if you like, move the foot up and down 3 times, like pressing on a pedal.

5. Find Your New Stretch

Key Phrase: We move slowly so you can "find a better way to move."

Opening Cue: Gentle seated stretches are a way to manage pain.

Cues:

1. Give yourself a few moments to create some simple stretches as you stand, sit, or lie down. You can move with me or find your own ways to stretch. (*Cue what you are doing as you move.*) Perhaps move your arms in a new way, one arm and then the other. Notice if you stretch your fingers wide. Then move both arms in a new way.
2. If you like, step your feet apart and move from side to side. Perhaps moving your hips in a circle is a new way to stretch today. Take your time as you move in a comfortable new way.
3. Now the suggestion is to take up space on the last stretch. If you like, put more effort into your breath in as you stretch your fingers and toes and arms. Take up space as you breathe and stretch in a comfortable way.
4. When you are ready, come back to standing or sitting tall.

6. Anytime, Anywhere Breath

Key Phrase: Long, slow breaths out can lower heart rate, lower blood pressure, and lower muscle tension.

Opening Cue: One way we can manage pain in real-time is by choosing how we breathe.

Cues: You can do the Anytime, Anywhere Breath even when talking with someone.

1. When you are ready, gently press one shoulder back... Then press the other shoulder back. If you like, place one hand on your leg in a way that is comfortable for you today.
2. Let's practice 5 breaths. The suggestion is to take long, slow breaths out. (**Variation 1.**)

As YOU breathe in, fingers press... As YOU breathe out, release. (*Say 2 times slowly.*)
Always breathe in a comfortable way.
On YOUR next breath in, fingers press... As YOU breathe out, release.
As YOU breathe in, fingers press... As YOU breathe out, release. (*Say 2 times slowly.*)

3. If you like, gently move the fingers on one hand or shake that hand... Then gently move the fingers on the other hand or shake that hand. (**Variation 2.**)
4. You may want to practice the Anytime, Anywhere Breath later, when you want to change how you are feeling.

Variations: (1) Press your fingers firmly or gently today. **Or** (2) Now if you like, use your other hand and practice saying it 3 times to yourself in your mind, since *you* are always with you. (*Say slowly during this time so you don't leave "dead air:" Don't rush your words... Don't rush your breath. Take your time with your words... Take your time with your breath.*)

C. Make a Plan

Opening Cue: Next time your start to feel pain or discomfort, you can have a 1- or 2-minute plan ready to go.

Cues:

1. The suggestion is to choose one breath we did today. We did Feel the Breath with Fingertip Press, Feel the Breath, Finger Stretch Breath, and the Anytime, Anywhere Breath. Long, slow breaths out *can* lower blood pressure. So now you have a 1-minute breath to do later when you want to change how you are feeling.
2. If you like, add one stretch to do again: perhaps the wide-legged add-on or Tip-to-Toe Stretch. You now have a 2-minute plan to manage your pain.
3. (See www.greentreeyoga.org/pain-management-resources for free downloads.)

D. Extras
1. Time Adjustments

Running Out of Time? When you notice you are running out of time, move ahead to the Anytime, Anywhere Breath. Then Make a Plan.

Too Much Time? After the Anytime, Anywhere Breath, stand again and repeat the Tip-to-Toe Stretch, wide-legged add-on, and Feel the Breath. Then take a seat to Make a Plan.

2. Theme Variation: The Pause
After you have done this practice several times, you can offer this idea at the beginning and mention it a few times during the practice:

> Today, you might want to notice if you pause between the breath in and the breath out. You don't need to change it, unless you want to play with pausing and noticing it.

III. GENTLY MOVING TOWARD A HEALTHIER SPINE (STANDING/SEATED)
Note: Before you teach, please review In Case You Missed It... (p.101)

A. Standing
1. Tip-to-Toe Stretch (photos on p.243)
Key Phrase: Lengthening the spine with the Tip-to-Toe Stretch is one way for you to move toward a healthier spine.

Opening Cue: As Moshé Feldenkrais said, "There isn't a right way to move; there is a better way to move."

Cues:

1. The suggestion is to stretch one arm to the side or overhead, fingers stretched wide in the Tip-to-Toe Stretch.
2. Then stretch the other arm, either to the side or overhead, fingers stretched wide.
3. Find your own rhythm as you stretch one arm and then the other. We move slowly so you can "find a better way to move" toward a healthier spine. (**Variation.**)
4. When you are ready, put your hands on your hips.
   If you like, lift one heel and press on your toes. Then lift the other heel and press on the toes. Let's create space between the toe joints two more times. (*Say 2 times slowly.*)

Variation: Today you may like to grasp one wrist as you stretch the other arm up toward the ceiling. Then grasp the other wrist and stretch up toward the ceiling.

2. Feel the Breath (photo on p.262)

Key Phrases: (1) Longer breaths in can be energizing. (2) Long, slow breaths out *can* lower heart rate, lower blood pressure, and lower muscle tension.

Opening Cue: One way we can manage pain in real-time is by choosing how we breathe.

Cues:

1. When you are ready, gently press one shoulder back... Then press the other shoulder back.
2. If you like, put one or both hands over your heart... Put one or both hands over your heart.
3. The suggestion is to practice 5 breaths. (**Variations.**)
   Feel the breath in... Feel the breath out. (*Say 2 times slowly.*)
   Always breathe in a comfortable way.
   Feel the breath in... Feel the breath out. (*Say 3 times slowly.*)
4. If you like, gently move the fingers on one hand or shake that hand...then gently move the fingers on the other hand or shake that hand.

Variations: (1) Today you may like to choose your breathing pattern: long breath in to energize or long breath out to lower blood pressure. **Or** (2) If you like, after you feel the breath in, pause long enough to notice the pause, then feel the breath out. **Or** (3) If you like, after you feel the breath out, pause long enough to notice the pause, then feel the breath in.

3. Side-to-Side (Lateral) Stretches (a/b)
A. CRESCENT STRETCH (PHOTO ON P.245)

Key Phrase: You can make any stretch as gentle or intense or you need today.

Opening Cue: Side-to-side (lateral) stretches as you are standing are two more ways for you to move toward a healthier spine.

Cues:

1. We always do both sides. When you are ready, put your hands on your hips. Then, lift or gently arc one shoulder. Today you may want to arc that arm overhead. If you like, stretch your fingers wide. When you are ready, gently lift and arc on the other side. That's 1 set. Find your own rhythm lifting and gently arcing one shoulder or one arm and then the other as you do 2 more sets. Notice if one side feels different than the other. (**Variation.**)
2. The suggestion is to finish by holding each stretch for 2 breaths. As you

lift and gently arc to one side, hold the stretch…but not your breath. Feel the breath in… Feel the breath out. (*Say 2 times slowly.*) When you are ready, lift and gently arc to the other side. Then hold the stretch…but not your breath. Feel the breath in… Feel the breath out. (*Say 2 times slowly.*)

3. Now if you like, gently move the fingers on one hand or shake that hand… Then gently move the fingers on the other hand or shake that hand.

Variation: Today you may like to grasp your wrist as you arc one arm overhead. Find your own rhythm as you move from side to side.

B. WIDE-LEGGED ADD-ON (PHOTOS ON P.245)

Key Phrase: Moving even half an inch or a few centimeters has benefits; it means muscles are not getting tighter.

Opening Cue: Gentle side-to-side (lateral) stretches as you stand and move toward a healthier spine can reduce pressure on nerves and joints.

Cues:

1. When you are ready, step your feet apart, hands on your hips as we do the wide-legged add-on. (**Variation.**)
2. In whatever way feels comfortable, move one hip to one side… Then move the other hip to the other side. We move slowly so you can "find a better way to move."
3. Today you may like to add lifting your shoulder in a gentle arc as you move to one side… Then lift the other shoulder in a gentle arc as you move the other hip to the side. Find your own rhythm as you move from side to side. Take your time as you move.
4. When you are ready, come back to standing tall. If you like, gently *stretch* the fingers on one hand or shake that hand… Then gently *stretch* the fingers or shake the other hand.

Variation: Today you may want to roll from the inside edges to the outside edges of your feet in a comfortable way… Roll from the inside to the outside edges in any way that is comfortable for you today.

4. Cat/Cow (Flex and Extend) (photos on p.242)

Key Phrase: Even small stretches have benefits.

Opening Cue: Gently bending the spine forward and back are two more ways to move toward spinal health.

Cues:

1. When you are ready, gently bend your knees...put your hands on your legs...and press your hips back. The suggestion is to practice this standing cat/cow stretch 3 times. Always move and breathe in a comfortable way.
2. As YOU breathe in...chin lifts...shoulders back...tailbone lifts. As YOU breathe out, chin tucks...shoulders forward...tailbone tucks.
3. Notice if you still have a slight bend in your knees. Always move in a comfortable way as we do 2 more sets. (*Say slowly 2 more times.*) (**Variation.**)

Variation: Stand with your knees slightly bent. Place your palms or gentle fists on your hips or back. Gently press one shoulder back... Then press the other shoulder back. Press your elbows back to create a supported backbend. The suggestion is to practice 3 breaths here. Feel the breath in... Feel the breath out. (*Say 3 times slowly.*) When you are ready, practice one more cat/cow stretch.

5. Twist: Ring the Bell (photos on p.249)

Key Phrase: We move slowly so we can "find a better way to move."

Opening Cue: Gentle twists can create more length in the spine.

Cues:

1. When you are ready, step your feet apart a comfortable distance. In any way that is comfortable for you today, gently swing your arms from the front to the back, tapping your low back...your midback...and your upper back as you move up and down your back.
2. If you like, change how you are holding your hands: now either "ring the bell" with an open palm or a gentle fist. Take your time with the stretch as you gently create length in your spine.

6. Tip-to-Toe Stretch (photos on p.243)

Key Phrase: Always move in a way that is comfortable for you today.

Opening Cue: Let's do the Tip-to-Toe Stretch again to gently lengthen the spine before we take a seat.

Cues:

1. As we did earlier, stretch one arm to the side or overhead in a comfortable way, fingers spread wide. Then stretch the other arm, fingers spread wide.
2. Find your own rhythm as you create length from tip-to-toe as you are

standing. Take your time with these stretches. When you are ready, come back to standing tall, arms by your sides.

B. Seated
1. Get Yourself Set Up
Key Phrases: (1) Anything we do seated, you can do standing or even lying down. (2) You can always find ways to move and to breathe with me.

Opening Cue: Sitting or standing with your shoulders gently pressed back can take pressure off your back.

Cues:

1. Give yourself a few moments to find a comfortable way to sit today, either on a folded blanket or on a chair.
2. Gently press one shoulder back... Then press the other shoulder back.
3. If you like, move from side to side as you settle into your seat. Perhaps move in a circle. Take your time as you move. You may want to circle even more slowly the other way.
4. Make any adjustments to make your seat more comfortable.

2. The Wave Breath (photos on p.262)
Key Phrases: (1) Long, slow breaths out *can* lower heart rate, lower blood pressure, and lower muscle tension. (2) Longer breaths in *can* be energizing.

Opening Cue: Noticing your breath can be the first step in managing how you breathe.

Cues:

1. Notice if your shoulders are still gently pressed back.
2. The suggestion is to take 5 breaths as we practice the Wave Breath.
   As YOU breathe in, hands lift (*palms up*)... As YOU breathe out, release (*palms down*). (*Say 2 times slowly.*)
   Always breathe in a comfortable way. On YOUR next breath in, hands lift... As YOU breathe out, release.
   As YOU breathe in, hands lift... As YOU breathe out, release. (*Say 2 times slowly.*)
3. If you like, gently move the fingers on one hand or shake that hand... Then gently move the fingers on the other hand or shake that hand.

3. Tip-to-Toe Stretch (photos on p.244)
Key Phrase: Different days, different stretches.

Opening Cue: There are many seated stretches that can move you toward a healthier spine.

Cues:

1. The suggestion is to do a seated Tip-to-Toe Stretch by stretching one arm to the side or overhead. If you like, stretch your fingers wide. Then stretch the other arm to the side or overhead, fingers stretched wide.
2. Find your own rhythm as you stretch one arm, fingers stretched wide... Then stretch the other arm, fingers spread wide.
3. Today you may like to stretch your toes as you stretch your fingers wide. Take your time with each stretch. When you are ready, arms by your sides.

4. Side-to-Side (Lateral) Stretches (a/b) (photos on pp.244, 254)
A. SHOULDER LIFT AND RELEASE

Key Phrase: We move slowly so you can "find a better way to move."

Opening Cue: Bending from side-to-side (lateral) stretches as you sit are two more ways for you to move toward a healthier spine.

Cues: The suggestion is to do 4 sets of this shoulder lift and release side-to-side stretch. With your arms by your sides, when you are ready, lift and gently arc one shoulder. Then lift and gently arc the other shoulder. That's 1 set. Find your own rhythm. (*Say 4 times slowly.*)

B. CRESCENT STRETCH

Key Phrase: Make the stretch as gentle or intense as you need today.

Opening Cue: You can continue lifting and gently arcing your shoulders, or today you may want a different stretch.

Cues:

1. We always do both sides. When you are ready, put your hands on your hips. Then either lift one shoulder in a gentle arc or arc that arm overhead in a comfortable way. If you like, wiggle your fingers. The suggestion is to find your own rhythm gently arcing one shoulder or one arm from side to side. Take your time with each stretch. (**Variation.**)
2. The suggestion is to now hold each stretch for 2 breaths. On one side, hold the stretch...but not your breath. Feel the breath in... Feel the breath out. (*Say 2 times slowly.*) When you are ready, on the other side, hold the stretch...but not your breath. Feel the breath in... Feel the breath out. (*Say 2 times slowly.*) When you are ready, come back to sitting tall.

Variation: Today you may like to grasp your wrist as you arc one arm overhead. Find your own rhythm as you move from side to side.

5. Cat/Cow (Flex and Extend) (photos on p.242)

Key Phrase: Different days, different stretches.

Opening Cue: Bending forward and back as you sit can create length in the spine.

Cues:

1. If you like, tap your *fingertips* on your legs. The suggestion is to practice seated cat/cow 2 times.
2. YOU breathe in, chin lifts…shoulders back…rock forward.
   As YOU breathe out, chin tucks…shoulders forward…rock back a comfortable distance. Always move and breathe in a comfortable way.
3. On YOUR next breath in, chin lifts…shoulders back…rock forward. As YOU breathe out chin tucks…shoulders forward…rock back a comfortable distance.
4. When you are ready, come back to sitting tall.
5. If you like, let's practice 2 more breaths. As YOU breathe in, press down on all your fingers and all your toes. As YOU breathe out, release. (*Say 2 times slowly.*)

6. Twists (a/b) (photos on p.254)

A. SHOULDER ROCK 'N ROLL

Key Phrase: Even small stretches have benefits.

Opening Cue: Gentle seated stretches can release some physical and emotional pain.

Cues:

1. Gently bend your elbows and stretch your fingers if that is comfortable for you today.
2. When you are ready, move one arm across the front, the other arm across the back as we practice shoulder Rock 'n Roll. Leading from the elbows if you like, now move the other arm across the front, and the other across the back. That's 1 set. Find your own rhythm as you practice 2 more sets. You can make each stretch as gentle or intense as you need today. Moving the arms from front to back in any way that feels comfortable… Finding your own rhythm as you move.

3. Now if you like, lead from the shoulders as you move from front to back. Practice as many sets as feels comfortable for you today... Moving the arms from front to back as slowly as you would like.
4. Now, the suggestion is to hold the stretch on each side for 2 breaths. As one shoulder moves across the front and the other across the back, hold the stretch...but not your breath. Feel the breath in... Feel the breath out. (*Say 2 times slowly.*)
5. Now as your other shoulder moves across the front and the other across the back, hold the stretch...but not your breath. Feel the breath in... Feel the breath out. (*Say 2 times slowly.*)
6. When you are ready, arms to your sides.

B. CLASSIC TWIST WITH CAT/COW (PHOTOS ON P.242)

Key Phrase: There is no place you are trying to go with a stretch.

Opening Cue: Let's do one more gentle twist to practice moving toward spinal health as we sit.

Cues:

1. Gently press one shoulder back... Then press the other shoulder back. If you like, tap your *fingertips* on your legs.
2. We always do both sides. On YOUR next breath in, press down on hands and feet. As YOU breathe out, bring hands around to one side. (**Variation.**)
3. Let's practice 4 breaths here. As YOU breathe in, hands press. As YOU breathe out, release the press. (*Say 4 times slowly.*)
4. When you are ready, come back to facing front. If you like, tap your *hands* on your legs.
   Before we do the other side, the suggestion is to practice seated cat/cow 2 times.
5. As YOU breathe in, chin lifts...shoulders back...rock forward.
   As YOU breathe out, chin tucks...shoulders forward...rock back a comfortable distance. Always move and breathe in a comfortable way.
6. On YOUR next breath in, chin lifts...shoulders back...rock forward. As YOU breathe out, chin tucks...shoulders forward...rock back a comfortable distance.
7. When you are ready, come back to sitting tall. (**Repeat on the other side.**)

Variation: When it feels comfortable to breathe in the twist, you may want to look forward for a full spinal twist. If you like, practice 4 more breaths here.

7. Anytime, Anywhere Breath

Key Phrase: Long, slow breaths out *can* lower heart rate, lower blood pressure, and lower muscle tension.

Opening Cue: You can interrupt your stress cycle by choosing how you breathe.

Cues: You can do the Anytime, Anywhere Breath even when talking with someone.

1. When you are ready, gently press one shoulder back... Then press the other shoulder back. If you like, place one hand on your leg in a way that is comfortable for you today.
2. Let's practice 5 breaths. The suggestion is to practice long, slow breaths out. (**Variation 1.**)
   As YOU breathe in, fingers press... As YOU breathe out, release. (*Say 2 times slowly.*)
   Always breathe in a comfortable way.
   On YOUR next breath in, fingers press... As YOU breathe out, release.
   As YOU breathe in, fingers press... As YOU breathe out, release. (*Say 2 times slowly.*)
3. If you like, gently move the fingers on one hand or shake that hand... Then gently move the fingers on the other hand or shake that hand. (**Variation 2.**)
4. You may want to practice the Anytime, Anywhere Breath later, when you want to change how you are feeling.

Variations: (1) Press your fingers firmly or gently today. **Or** (2) Now if you like, use your other hand and practice saying it 3 times to yourself in your mind, since *you* are always with you. (*Say slowly during this time so there is no "dead air:" Don't rush your words... Don't rush your breath. Take your time with your words... Take your time with your breath.*)

C. Make a Plan

Opening Cue: Next time you start to feel pain or discomfort, you can have a 1- to 2-minute plan ready to go.

Cues:

1. The suggestion is to choose one breath we did today: we did Feel the Breath, the Wave Breath, and the Anytime, Anywhere Breath. Long, slow breaths out *can* lower blood pressure. So now you have a 1-minute breath to do later when you want to change how you are feeling.

2. If you like, add one stretch to do again. Perhaps include Tip-to-Toe Stretch or shoulder Rock 'n Roll. You now have a 2-minute plan to manage your pain.
3. (See www.greentreeyoga.org/pain-management-resources for free downloads.)

D. Extras
1. Time Adjustments

Running Out of Time? When you notice you are running out of time, move ahead to the Anytime, Anywhere Breath. Then Make a Plan.

Too Much Time? After the Anytime, Anywhere Breath, stand again and repeat the Tip-to-Toe Stretch, crescent stretch, and Feel the Breath. Then take a seat to Make a Plan.

2. Theme Variation: Savor the Stretch

After you have done this practice several times, you can offer this idea at the beginning and mention it a few times during the practice:

> Today, you might want to move even more slowly than in our last practice. Give yourself a moment to Savor the Stretch.

IV. STRETCH AND BREATHE (SEATED)
Note: Before you teach, please review In Case You Missed It... (p.101)

A. Seated
1. Get Yourself Set Up
Key Phrases: (1) Anything we do seated, you can do standing or even lying down. (2) You can always find ways to move and to breathe with me.

Opening Cue: Sitting or standing with your shoulders gently pressed back can take pressure off your back.

Cues:

1. Give yourself a few moments to find a comfortable way to sit today, either on a folded blanket or on a chair.
2. Gently press one shoulder back... Then press the other shoulder back.
3. If you like, move from side to side as you settle into your seat. Perhaps move in a circle. Take your time as you move. You may want to circle the other way even more slowly.
4. Make any adjustments to make your seat more comfortable.

2. Tip-to-Toe Stretch (photos on p.244)
Key Phrase: Different days, different stretches.

Opening Cue: We move slowly to practice "finding a better way to move" as we sit.

Cues:

1. The suggestion is to stretch one arm to the side or overhead, fingers stretched wide in the seated Tip-to-Toe Stretch.
2. When you are ready, stretch the other arm, either to the side or overhead, fingers stretched wide, gently lengthening the spine as you move.
3. Find your own rhythm as you stretch one arm and then the other. Take your time with each stretch. Perhaps stretch your toes as you stretch your fingers. (**Variation.**)

Variation: Either lift and gently arc one shoulder or arc that arm overhead in a comfortable way in crescent stretch. Then lift and gently arc the other shoulder or arc that arm in a comfortable way.

3. Feel the Breath
Key Phrase: Longer breaths in *can* be energizing.

Opening Cue: One way we can manage pain in real-time is by choosing how we breathe.

Cues:

1. When you are ready, gently press one shoulder back... Then press the other shoulder back.
2. If you like, put one or both hands over your heart... Put one or both hands over your heart.
3. The suggestion is to practice 5 breaths. (**Variation 1 or 2.**)
   Feel the breath in... Feel the breath out. (*Say 2 times slowly.*)
   Always breathe in a comfortable way.
   Feel the breath in... Feel the breath out. (*Say 3 times slowly.*)
4. If you like, gently move the fingers on one hand or shake that hand... Then gently move the fingers on the other hand or shake that hand.

Variations: (1) If you like, after you feel the breath in, pause long enough to notice the pause... Then feel the breath out... **Or** (2) If you like, after you feel the breath out, pause long enough to notice the pause, then feel the breath in...

4. 1-2-3 Shoulder Stretch (photos on p.254)

Key Phrases: (1) Even small stretches have benefits. (2) Long, slow breaths out *can* lower blood pressure.

Opening Cue: The suggestion is to practice 1-2-3 Shoulder Stretch 3 times.

Cues:

1. Gently bend your elbows with fingers stretched wide if that is comfortable for you today.
2. As YOU breathe in, shoulders and elbows press back... That's 1. As YOU breathe out, shoulders and elbows press forward... That's 2. And release... That's 3. And that's 1 set. You can make each stretch as gentle or intense as you need today.
3. The suggestion is to practice 2 more sets of 1-2-3 Shoulder Stretch. (*Say slowly 2 more times.*)

5. #4 Stretch (a/b/c) (photos on p.251)
A. #4 FLOW

Key Phrase: Always move in a comfortable way.

Opening Cue: Gentle hip stretches can help manage pain.

Cues:

1. We always do both sides. When you are ready, cross one ankle over your other leg in the #4 stretch. Support your knee with your hands. Pull your toes toward your shin.
2. Gently press one shoulder back... Then press the other shoulder back.
3. The suggestion is to hold your knee steady as you gently press your knee against your hands. Your knee doesn't move. If you like, practice 3 breaths. Feel the breath in... Feel the breath out. (*Say 3 times slowly.*)
4. When you are ready, release your hands and gently let your knee press down—it may be half an inch or a few centimeters. Notice if your toes are still pressing up toward your shin. (**Variation.**)

Variation: If you like, slide your hands back on the chair or floor. Gently press one shoulder back... Then press the other shoulder back. Let's practice 3 breaths as you find your own rhythm. As YOU breathe in, release forward a comfortable distance... As YOU breathe out, sit up, shoulders still gently pressing back. (*Say 3 times slowly.*)

B. #4 TWIST

Key Phrase: You can always adjust the twist; you are never stuck.

Opening Cue: A gentle twist can stretch the piriformis muscle and help manage sciatic or low back pain.

Cues:

1. When you are ready, create your twist by bringing your hands across to the side. Perhaps press one hand on the ball of your foot.
2. Notice if this is a comfortable place to breathe. Make any adjustments. (**Variation.**)
3. The suggestion is to find your own rhythm as you practice 4 breaths. As YOU breathe in, gently press down on your hands… As YOU breathe out, release. (*Say slowly 4 times.*)
4. When you are ready, come back to facing the front, feet on the floor.

Variation: You may want to look forward as you create a full spinal twist.

C. CAT/COW

Key Phrase: Today you may want to practice long, slow breaths out.

Opening Cue: Gentle stretching can help reduce both emotional and physical pain.

Cues:

1. If you like, tap your *fingertips* on your legs. The suggestion is to practice seated cat/cow 2 times.
2. As YOU breathe in, chin lifts…shoulders back…rock forward. As YOU breathe out, chin tucks…shoulders forward…rock back a comfortable distance. Always move and breathe in a comfortable way.
3. On YOUR next breath in, chin lifts…shoulders back…rock forward. As YOU breathe out, chin tucks…shoulders forward…rock back a comfortable distance.
4. When you are ready, come back to sitting tall. (**Repeat a/b/c on the other side.**)

6. Finger Stretch Breath

Key Phrase: Long, slow breaths out *can* lower heart rate, lower blood pressure, and lower muscle tension.

Opening Cue: One way we can manage pain in real-time is by choosing how we breathe.

Cues: In Finger Stretch Breath, the suggestion is to stretch your fingers half an inch or a few centimeters. (**Variations.**)

1. When you are ready, gently press one shoulder back… Then press the other shoulder back.
2. If you like, let's practice 5 breaths. As YOU breathe in, fingers stretch… As YOU breathe out, release. (*Say 2 times slowly.*)
Always breathe in a comfortable way.
On YOUR next breath in, fingers stretch… As YOU breathe out, release. As YOU breathe in, fingers stretch… As YOU breathe out, release. (*Say 2 times slowly.*)
3. If you like, gently move the fingers on one hand or shake that hand… Then gently move the fingers on the other hand or shake that hand.

Variations: (1) Stretch just enough to notice the stretch. **Or** (2) Stretch your fingers as wide as you would like today. **Or** (3) Perhaps stretch your fingers in a different way today.

7. Eagle Flow (a/b/c) (photos on p.241)

A. EAGLE WRAP

Key Phrases: (1) Today you may want to find a new way to stretch. (2) Different days, different stretches.

Opening Cue: Let's gently stretch the outer hip muscles and the glutes.

Cues:

1. When you are ready, gently press one shoulder back… Then press the other shoulder back.
2. We always do both sides. If you like, cross one leg over the other. A different way is to wrap your foot around the other leg. (**Variation.**)
3. Press your left leg to the left while your press your right leg to the right. The suggestion is to keep pressing in a comfortable way as we practice 4 breaths. Feel the breath in… Feel the breath out. (*Say 4 times slowly.*)

Variation: If you like, slide your hands back on the chair or floor. Gently press one shoulder back… Then press the other shoulder back. Let's practice 3 breaths as you find your own rhythm. As YOU breathe in, release forward a comfortable distance… As YOU breathe out, sit up, shoulders still gently pressing back. (*Say 3 times slowly.*)

B. EAGLE WRAP IN A TWIST

Key Phrase: You can always adjust the twist; you are never stuck.

Opening Cue: This gentle twist can stretch the outer hip and spinal muscles.

Cues:

1. Notice which leg is on top. When you are ready, create your twist by bringing both hands to that side. (*Left leg on top, twist to the left.*)
2. Make any adjustments as you find a comfortable place to practice 4 breaths. (**Variation.**) Feel the breath in... Feel the breath out. (*Say 2 times slowly.*)
3. Still in your twist, you may want to look forward to create a full spinal twist. Feel the breath in... Feel the breath out. (*Say 2 times slowly.*)
4. When you are ready, come back to facing front, two feet on the floor.

Variation: Find your own rhythm: As YOU breathe in, hands press... As YOU breathe out, release the press. (*Say 4 times slowly.*)

C. CAT/COW

Key Phrase: Today you may want to practice long, slow breaths out.

Opening Cue: Let's gently stretch the muscles along the front and the back of the spine.

Cues:

1. If you like, tap your *fingertips* on your legs. The suggestion is to practice seated cat/cow 2 times.
2. As YOU breathe in, chin lifts...shoulders back...rock forward.
3. As YOU breathe out, chin tucks...shoulders forward...rock back a comfortable distance. Always move and breathe in a comfortable way.
4. On YOUR next breath in, chin lifts...shoulders back...rock forward. As YOU breathe out, chin tucks...shoulders forward...rock back a comfortable distance.
5. When you are ready, come back to sitting tall. (**Repeat a/b/c on the other side.**)

8. Fancy Footwork (photos on p.000 [AQ])

Key Phrase: Always move in a comfortable way.

Opening Cue: Stretching the muscles and connective tissue in the feet and ankles as you sit can ease pressure on joints and improve circulation.

Cues:

1. When you are ready, lift your leg a comfortable distance and put your hands around your shin or the back of your leg.

2. Gently press one shoulder back... Then press the other shoulder back.
3. If you like, slowly move this foot in a circle... Then circle the other way. (**Variation.**)
4. Give yourself a moment to move your foot in a new way, taking your time with the stretch.
5. If you like, stretch all your toes 3 times. As YOU breathe in, stretch your toes... As YOU breathe out, release. (*Say 3 times slowly.*) (**Repeat on the other side.**)

Variation: If you like, slowly move your big toe as if writing the name of your favorite place (food, animal...).

9. Quads and Psoas Stretch with Cat/Cow (photos on p.257)

Key Phrase: Small stretches and even visualizing a stretch have benefits.

Opening Cue: You can gently stretch two large muscles as you sit—the psoas muscle is the thick front hip flexor and the quadriceps are the large front leg muscles from the knee to the hip bone.

Cues:

1. The suggestion is to sit to one side of your chair. When you are ready, create a comfortable quads stretch by bending your knee and moving your leg back. Today you may hold your ankle or pant leg.
2. If you like, practice 3 breaths here. Feel the breath in... Feel the breath out. (*Say 3 times slowly.*)
3. When you are ready, still holding your ankle or pant leg if you like, lift your leg back and to the side for the psoas stretch. Move slowly so you can "find a better way to move." If you like, practice 3 breaths here. Feel the breath in... Feel the breath out. (*Say 3 times slowly.*)
4. When you are ready, come back to sitting tall. If you like, tap your *hands* on your legs.
5. The suggestion is to practice seated cat/cow 2 times.
6. As YOU breathe in, chin lifts...shoulders back...rock forward.
   As YOU breathe out, chin tucks...shoulders forward...rock back a comfortable distance. Always move and breathe in a comfortable way.
7. On YOUR next breath in, chin lifts...shoulders back...rock forward. As YOU breathe out, chin tucks...shoulders forward...rock back a comfortable distance. (**Repeat on the other side.**)
8. When you are ready, come back to sitting tall.

10. Neck and Shoulder Suite (a/b/c) (photos on p.255)

A. NECK MASSAGE

Key Phrase: Always move in a way that is comfortable for you today.

Opening Cue: Gently massaging muscles as you sit can reduce physical and emotional tension.

Cues:

1. The suggestion is to use one hand to massage the back of your neck, or if it's more comfortable for you today, the fronts of your shoulders. **(Variation.)**
2. Today you may want to: (*Slowly cue as you do each one.*)
   a. Use one or both hands.
   b. Gently tuck your chin and move your chin from side to side as you massage.
   c. Massage the base of your neck/top of your back.
   d. Gently lift and lower your chin as you massage.

Variation: Use a gentle or firm massage in a way that feels comfortable for you today.

B. CHIN LIFTS AND PENDULUM

Key Phrases: (1) You may be moving half an inch or a few centimeters, and that has benefits. (2) Some days, visualizing the stretch may be more helpful.

Opening Cue: The head weighs about 10 pounds or 4.5 kilograms. Gently stretching neck muscles can relieve some tension and pain.

Cues:

1. The suggestion is to practice chin lifts 3 times. As YOU breathe in, chin slowly lifts... As YOU breathe out, chin slowly releases. (*Say slowly 3 times.*)
2. With your chin still released, slowly move your chin from side to side, like a pendulum. Take your time with each slow stretch. When you are ready, come back to sitting tall.

C. NECK AND SHOULDER STRETCHES (PHOTOS ON P.255)

Key Phrase: You can change how you are stretching any time; you are never stuck.

Opening Cue: Gently stretching muscles around the neck and shoulders as you sit can reduce some neck and back pain.

Cues:

1. We always do both sides. The suggestion is to gently release your *left* ear toward your *left* shoulder. Moving even half an inch or a few centimeters has benefits.
2. When you are ready, move your *right* shoulder, practicing each of these slow stretches 3 times:
    a. Press your shoulder forward... Then press it back. (*Say 3 times slowly.*)
    b. As YOU breathe in, lift that shoulder... As YOU breathe out, press that shoulder down as firmly as is comfortable for you today. If you like, hold this press for 2 more breaths. Hold the press...but not your breath. Feel the breath in... Feel the breath out. (*Say 2 times slowly.*) **(Repeat 2 more times.)**
    c. Now roll this shoulder forward 3 times in a comfortable way. Take your time with this slow stretch. When you are ready, roll this shoulder back 3 times. Again, take your time as you "find a better way to move."
3. When you are ready, come back to sitting tall. If you like, let's practice 2 more chin lifts. On YOUR breath in, chin slowly lifts... On YOUR breath out, chin slowly releases. (*Say 2 times slowly.*) **(Repeat #1-3 on the other side.)**

11. Feel the Breath with Fingertip Press

Key Phrase: Long, slow breaths in *can* be energizing.

Opening Cue: Noticing your breath can be a first step in managing how you breathe.

Cues:

1. When you are ready, gently press one shoulder back... Then press the other shoulder back.
2. If you like, put one or both hands over your heart... Put one or both hands over your heart.
3. Let's practice 5 breaths. Feel the breath in, fingertips press... Feel the breath out, release the press. (*Say 2 times slowly.*)
   Always breathe in a comfortable way.
   Feel the breath in, fingertips press... Feel the breath out, release. (*Say 3 times slowly.*)
4. If you like, gently move the fingers on one hand or shake that hand... Then gently move the fingers on the other hand or shake that hand.

B. Make a Plan

Opening Cue: Next time you start to feel pain or discomfort, you can have a 1- to 2-minute plan ready to go.

Cues:

1. The suggestion is to choose one breath we did today. We did Feel the Breath, Finger Stretch Breath, and Feel the Breath with fingertip press. Long, slow breaths out *can* lower blood pressure. So now you have a 1-minute breath to do later when you want to change how you are feeling.
2. If you like, add one stretch to do again. Perhaps include Tip-to-Toe Stretch or the #4 stretches. You now have a 2-minute plan to manage your pain.
3. (See www.greentreeyoga.org/pain-management-resources for free downloads.)

C. Extras

1. Time Adjustments

Running Out of Time? When you notice you are running out of time, move ahead to Feel the Breath with fingertip press. Then Make a Plan.

Too Much Time? After Feel the Breath with fingertip press, repeat seated Tip-to-Toe Stretch, 1-2-3 Shoulder Stretch, and cat/cow. Then find a comfortable seat to Make a Plan.

2. Theme Variation: Stretch the Toes

After you have done this practice several times, you can offer this idea at the beginning and mention it a few times during the practice:

> Today as we stretch and breathe, perhaps add stretching your toes on any breath in and releasing your toes on any breath out.

V. NEW WAYS TO STRETCH AND BREATHE (KNEELING/SEATED)

Note: Before you teach, please review In Case You Missed It... (p.101)

A. Kneel 'n Stretch (photos on p.256)
1. Get Yourself Set Up
Key Phrase: Different days, different stretches.

Opening Cues: "Finding a better way to move" can be a key to managing pain. When we do not move, muscles can tighten and press on nerves and joints.

Cues:

1. To get yourself set up to do Kneel 'n Stretch, the suggestion is to kneel on a folded mat or pillow with your fingers interlaced and forearms resting on a padded chair seat. Lining your elbows up with your shoulders can protect your shoulder joints.
2. Gently press one shoulder back... Then press the other shoulder back.
3. Let's practice 3 breaths. As YOU breathe in, hands gently press... As YOU breathe out, hips press back. (*Say 3 times slowly.*)
4. Now make any adjustments as you "find a better way to move."

2. Hip Rock 'n Roll
Key Phrase: Even small stretches have benefits.

Opening Cue: Let's gently stretch more muscles in the back and legs with hip Rock 'n Roll.

Cues:

1. When you are ready, tuck your tailbone...and then lift your tailbone... finding your own rhythm.
2. Notice how the stretch changes as you move. Take your time as you tuck your tailbone and then lift your tailbone in any way that feels comfortable for you today.
3. On your last set, when you tuck your tailbone, if you like, hold the stretch...but not your breath. Let's practice 2 breaths. Feel the breath in... Feel the breath out. (*Say 2 times slowly.*)
4. When you are ready, lift your tailbone again. If you like, hold the stretch... but not the breath. Feel the breath in... Feel the breath out. (*Say 2 times slowly.*)
5. Now gently press your hips back as we do Feel the Breath with fingertip press.

3. Feel the Breath with Fingertip Press
Opening Cue: You can interrupt your stress cycle by choosing how you breathe.

Cues:

1. When you are ready, still in Kneel 'n Stretch, gently press one shoulder back… Then press the other shoulder back.
2. Let's practice 3 breaths. Feel the breath in, fingertips press… Feel the breath out, release the press. (*Say 3 times slowly.*)

4. Psoas and Glutes Stretch

Key Phrases: (1) We move slowly so you can "find a better way to move." (2) Gently stretching and releasing these hip muscles can reduce pain.

Opening Cue: The psoas muscles are large muscles in the front of the hip. The glutes are the three muscles in the back of the hip bone.

Cues:

1. We always do both sides. When you are ready, extend one leg back any distance. Today you may want to lift that leg a comfortable distance. Then tuck your chin and draw that knee a comfortable distance toward your nose.
2. The suggestion is to do this stretch 3 times on each side.
3. On YOUR breath in, press one leg back and perhaps up…on YOUR breath in, chin tucks…leg tucks. (*Say 3 times slowly on each side.*)

5. Wide Knee Stretches

Key Phrase: Moving even half an inch or a few centimeters has benefits; it means muscles are not getting tighter.

Opening Cue: We move slowly so you can practice "finding a better way to move."

Cues:

1. When you are ready, move your knees apart a comfortable distance.
2. Gently move one hip to one side… Then move the other hip toward the other side.
3. If you like, find a new way to move. Perhaps today gently circling your hips feels like a comfortable stretch.
4. The suggestion is to find your own rhythm as you move. Notice how the stretch changes as you move.
5. Perhaps hold one stretch for 2 breaths. Feel the breath in… Feel the breath out. (*Say 2 times slowly.*) Then hold a different stretch for 2 breaths. Feel the breath in… Feel the breath out. (*Say 2 times slowly.*)

THIRTY-MINUTE PRACTICES

6. When you are ready, bring your knees back under your hips.

6. Quads and Psoas Stretches/Twist (photos on p.257)

Key Phrase: You can always change how you are moving; you are never stuck.

Opening Cue: You can gently stretch two large muscles now. The quadriceps are the large muscles from the knee to the hip bone. The psoas muscle is the thick front hip flexor.

Cues:

1. The suggestion is to place one forearm across the chair seat. When you are ready, create a comfortable quads stretch. Bend your knee a comfortable distance on the opposite side and press your leg back. Today you may hold your ankle or pant leg. If you like, practice 3 breaths here. Feel the breath in... Feel the breath out. (*Say 3 times slowly.*)
2. For the psoas stretch, now lift your knee out to the side and back a comfortable distance. Let's practice 3 breaths here. Feel the breath in... Feel the breath out. (*Say 3 times slowly.*)
3. When you are ready, release your knee.
4. Now for the gentle twist on the same side. Place your palm or a gentle fist on the side or back of your hip. If you like, look over that shoulder. The suggestion is to practice 3 breaths to gently lengthen the spine. Feel the breath in... Feel the breath out. (*Say 3 times slowly.*) (**Repeat on the other side.**)

7. Hip Rock 'n Roll (Repeat #2)

8. Cat/Cow (photos on p.000 [AQ])

Key Phrase: Take your time with each slow stretch.

Opening Cue: A cat/cow can give you more spinal stretch as we complete this flow.

Cues:

1. When you are ready, the suggestion is to gently lift your chin a comfortable distance...and lift your tailbone. Then gently tuck your chin...and tuck your tailbone. If you like, let's practice 2 more cat/cow stretches. Always move and breathe in a comfortable way.
2. On YOUR next breath in, chin lifts...tailbone lifts. As YOU breathe out, chin tucks...tailbone tucks.

3. Find your own rhythm as you breathe and move in another cat/cow stretch. (**Repeat #2.**)
4. Now if you like, create a side stretch by moving your hips to one side and then looking back, as if you see a tail wagging. The suggestion is to practice 2 breaths here. Feel the breath in… Feel the breath out. (*Say 2 times slowly.*) (**Repeat side stretch on the other side.**)
5. If you like, practice another cat/cow stretch before we stretch the other side. (**Repeat #1.**)

B. Seated
1. Get Yourself Set Up
Key Phrases: (1) Anything we do seated, you can do standing or even lying down. (2) You can always find ways to move and to breathe with me.

Opening Cue: Sitting or standing with your shoulders gently pressed back can take pressure off your back.

Cues:

1. Give yourself a few moments to find a comfortable way to sit today, either on a folded blanket or on a chair.
2. Gently press one shoulder back… Then press the other shoulder back.
3. If you like, move from side to side as you settle into your seat. Perhaps move in a circle. Take your time as you move. You may want to circle even more slowly the other way.
4. Make any adjustments for a more comfortable seat.

2. Tip-to-Toe Stretch (photos on p.244)
Key Phrase: Different days, different stretches.

Opening Cue: We move slowly as we sit to practice "finding a better way to move."

Cues:

1. When you are ready, stretch one arm to the side or overhead, fingers stretched wide in the Tip-to-Toe Stretch.
2. Then stretch the other arm, either to the side or overhead, fingers stretched wide, gently lengthening the spine as you move.
3. Find your own rhythm as you stretch one arm and then the other.
4. Perhaps stretch your toes as you stretch your fingers. Again, take your time "finding a better way to move."

3. Physiological Sigh

Key Phrase: Practicing the physiological sigh 2 or 3 times can help lower carbon dioxide levels in the blood, which can lower anxiety.

Opening Cue: You can interrupt your stress cycle by choosing how you breathe.

Cues:

1. When you are ready, gently press one shoulder back... Then press the other shoulder back.
2. Let's practice once. Always move and breathe in a comfortable way. When you are ready, practice a deep breath in and stretch your fingers wide. Then breathe in more; perhaps stretch your fingers a little more. Hold that breath as long as you like...when you are ready, SIGH it out, fingers release. The suggestion is to practice 2 more times. (*Say 2 more times.*)
3. The Physiological Sigh is a way to practice lowering your anxiety levels in 2 or 3 breaths.
4. If you like, gently move the fingers on one hand or shake that hand... Then gently move the fingers on the other hand or shake that hand.

4. Shoulder Rolls (photos on p.254)

Key Phrase: Today you may want to practice long breaths out.

Opening Cue: Long breaths out *can* reduce muscle tension.

Cues:

1. If you like, let's practice 3 shoulder rolls forward and 3 shoulder rolls back. As YOU breathe in, shoulders lift... As YOU breathe out, shoulders roll forward and down.
   Always move in a comfortable way. (*Say 3 times slowly.*)
2. Now 3 back. As YOU breathe in, shoulders lift... As YOU breathe out, shoulders roll back and down. (*Say 3 times slowly.*)

Variations: (1) After one roll: if you like, move even more slowly on the next two rolls. **Or** (2) After two rolls: if you like, stop halfway down this last roll. Hold the stretch...but not your breath.

5. Find a New Shoulder Stretch

Key Phrase: Moving slowly allows you to practice "finding a better way to move."

Opening Cue: Gentle stretches can help reduce both physical and emotional pain.

Cues: Give yourself a few moments to create some simple stretches. You can move with me or find your own ways to stretch. (*Cue what you are doing as you move.*)

6. Fancy Footwork (photos on pp.260–1)

Key Phrase: Always move in a comfortable way.

Opening Cue: Stretching the muscles and connective tissue in the feet and ankles as you sit can ease pressure on joints and improve circulation.

Cues:

1. When you are ready, lift your leg a comfortable distance and put your hands around your shin (or back of your leg).
2. Gently press one shoulder back… Then press the other shoulder back to take stress off your back.
3. If you like, slowly move this foot in a circle… Then circle the other way. (**Variation.**)
4. Give yourself a few moments to move your foot in a new way, taking your time with the slow stretch.
5. If you like, stretch all your toes 3 times. As YOU breathe in, stretch your toes… As YOU breathe out, release. (*Say 3 times slowly.*) (**Repeat on the other side.**)

Variation: If you like, slowly move your big toe as if writing the name of your favorite place (food, animal…).

7. Neck and Shoulder Suite (a/b/c) (photos on p.255)

A. NECK MASSAGE

Key Phrase: Even small stretches have benefits.

Opening Cue: Gently massaging muscles as you sit can reduce physical and emotional tension.

Cues:

1. The suggestion is to use one hand to massage the back of your neck, or if it's more comfortable for you today, the fronts of your shoulders. (**Variation.**)

2. Today you may want to: (*Slowly cue as you do each one.*)
   a. Use one or both hands.
   b. Gently tuck your chin and move your chin from side to side as you massage.
   c. Massage the base of your neck/top of your back.
   d. Gently lift and lower your chin as you massage.

Variation: Use a gentle or firm massage in a way that feels comfortable for you today.

B. CHIN LIFTS AND PENDULUM

Key Phrases: (1) You may be moving half an inch or a few centimeters, and that has benefits. (2) Some days, visualizing the stretch may be more helpful.

Opening Cue: The head weighs about 10 pounds or 4.5 kilograms. Gently stretching neck muscles can relieve some tension and pain.

Cues:

1. The suggestion is to practice this *slow* stretch 3 times. As YOU breathe in, chin slowly lifts... As YOU breathe out, chin slowly releases. (*Say slowly 3 times.*)
2. With your chin still released, slowly move your chin from side to side, like a pendulum. Take your time with each slow stretch.

C. NECK AND SHOULDER STRETCHES

Key Phrase: You can change how you are stretching any time; you are never stuck.

Opening Cue: Gently stretching muscles around the neck and shoulders as you sit can reduce some neck and back pain.

Cues:

1. We always do both sides. The suggestion is to gently release your *left* ear toward your *left* shoulder. Moving even half an inch or a few centimeters has benefit.
2. When you are ready, move your *right* shoulder, practicing each of these slow stretches 3 times:
   a. Press your shoulder forward... Then press it back. (*Say 3 times slowly.*)
   b. As YOU breathe in, lift that shoulder... As YOU breathe out, press that shoulder down as firmly as is comfortable for you today. If you

like, hold this press for 2 more breaths. Hold the press…but not your breath. Feel the breath in… Feel the breath out. (*Say 2 times slowly.*) (**Repeat 2 more times.**)
   c. Now roll this shoulder forward 3 times in a comfortable way. Take your time with this slow stretch. When you are ready, roll this shoulder back 3 times. Again, take your time as you "find a better way to move."
3. When you are ready, come back to sitting tall. If you like, let's practice 2 more chin lifts. On YOUR breath in, chin slowly lifts… On YOUR breath out, chin slowly releases. (*Say 2 times slowly.*) (**Repeat #1–3 on the other side.**)

8. Feel the Breath

Key Phrases: (1) Long, slow breaths out *can* lower blood pressure. (2) Longer breaths in *can* be energizing.

Opening Cue: Noticing your breath can be the first step in managing how you breathe.

Cues:

1. When you are ready, gently press one shoulder back… Then press the other shoulder back.
2. If you like, put one or both hands over your heart… Put one or both hands over your heart.
3. The suggestion is to practice 5 breaths. (**Variation.**)
   Feel the breath in… Feel the breath out. (*Say 2 times slowly.*)
   Always breathe in a comfortable way.
   Feel the breath in… Feel the breath out. (*Say 3 times slowly.*)
4. If you like, gently move the fingers on one hand or shake that hand… Then gently move the fingers on the other hand or shake that hand.

Variation: Today you may want to choose a breathing pattern: long breath in *can* energize, long breath out *can* lower blood pressure. Always breathe in a comfortable way.

C. Make a Plan

Opening Cue: Next time you start to feel pain or discomfort, you can have a 1- to 2-minute plan ready to go.

Cues:

1. The suggestion is to choose one breath we did today. We did Feel the Breath, Feel the Breath with fingertip press, and the physiological sigh. Long, slow breaths out *can* lower blood pressure. So now you have a 1-minute breath to do later when you want to change how you are feeling.
2. If you like, add one stretch to do again. Perhaps include shoulder rolls or Kneel 'n Stretch. You now have a 2-minute plan to manage your pain.
3. (See www.greentreeyoga.org/pain-management-resources for free downloads.)

D. Extras
1. Time Adjustments

Running Out of Time? When you notice you are running out of time, move ahead to Feel the Breath and Make a Plan.

Too Much Time? After Feel the Breath, repeat seated Tip-to-Toe Stretch, shoulder rolls, and Feel the Breath with fingertip press.

2. Theme Variation: The Pause (Take 2)

After you have done this practice several times, you can offer this idea at the beginning and mention it a few times during the practice:

> Today, you might want to notice if you pause after the breath out. You don't need to change it, unless you want to play with pausing and noticing it.

VI. SUPPORTED STRETCH AND RESTORE (LYING DOWN/SEATED)

Note: Before teaching, please review In Case You Missed It... (p.101)

A. Lying Down with Supported Spine
1. Get Yourself Set Up (photo on p.258)

Key Phrases: (1) Anything we do lying down, you can do seated or standing. (2) You can always find ways to move and to breathe with me.

Opening Cue: Major muscles that usually work to hold us up can release when we lie down.

Cues: Give yourself a few moments to get yourself set up. You can make adjustments; you are never stuck.

1. As you sit on the floor, you may want a rolled-up blanket, towel, or mat under your knees before you lie back.
2. One suggestion is to place a rolled-up mat or blanket roll along your spine with support for your head.

2. Feel the Breath
Key Phrase: Long, slow breaths out *can* lower heart rate, lower blood pressure, and lower muscle tension.

Opening Cue: One way we can manage pain in real-time is by choosing how we breathe.

Cues:

1. When you are ready, gently press one shoulder back... Then press the other shoulder back.
2. If you like, put one or both hands over your heart... Put one or both hands over your heart.
3. The suggestion is to take 5 breaths. Today you may like to practice long breaths out. (**Variation.**)
   Feel the breath in... Feel the breath out. (*Say 2 times slowly.*)
   Always breathe in a comfortable way.
   Feel the breath in... Feel the breath out. (*Say 3 times slowly.*)
4. If you like, gently move the fingers on one hand or shake that hand...then gently move the fingers on the other hand or shake that hand.

Variation: If you like, after you feel the breath out, pause long enough to notice the pause, then feel the breath in.

3. 1-2-3 Shoulder Stretch (photos on p.254)
Key Phrases: (1) Even small stretches have benefits. (2) Long, slow breaths out *can* lower blood pressure.

Opening Cue: The suggestion is to practice 1-2-3 Shoulder Stretch 3 times.

Cues:

1. Gently bend your elbows with fingers stretched wide if that is comfortable for you today.

2. As YOU breathe in, shoulders and elbows press back... That's 1.
   As YOU breathe out, shoulders and elbows press forward... That's 2.
   And release... That's 3. And that's 1 set. You can make each stretch as gentle or intense as you need today.
3. The suggestion is to practice 2 more sets of 1-2-3 Shoulder Stretch. (*Say slowly 2 more times.*)

4. Gentle Twist with Knees (photos on p.258)

Key Phrases: (1) We move slowly so we have time "to find a better way to move." (2) There is no place you are trying to go with the stretch.

Opening Cue: A gentle twist can create space between the spinal bones and stretch the outer hip muscles.

Cues:

1. You may want to move the rolled-up mat or blanket but keep a small roll (washcloth or towel) under your neck for support.
2. When you are ready, put your feet on the floor under your knees. Extend your arms, palms up or down, in a comfortable way.
3. Slowly move your knees from side to side, noticing what feels like a comfortable stretch today.
4. You can add to the stretch by crossing one knee over the other. We always do both sides. (**Variation.**) Continue to move slowly from side to side.
5. The suggestion is to find one gentle twist to hold. Hold the stretch...but not the breath. Let's take 2 breaths. Feel the breath in... Feel the breath out. (*Say 2 times slowly.*)
6. If you like, cross your knees the other way and find your own rhythm as you move.
7. Again, the suggestion is to find one gentle twist to hold. Hold the stretch...but not the breath. Let's take 2 breaths. Feel the breath in... Feel the breath out. (*Say 2 times slowly.*)
8. When you are ready, uncross your legs, pull them in, and rock from side to side. (**Repeat on the other side.**)

Variation: If you like, slowly move your knees to one side and look the opposite way as you create a full spinal twist.

5. Bridge Flow (a/b/c) (photos on p.259)

A. RAISING YOUR HEART

Key Phrase: Use the pieces of the stretch that feel comfortable for you today.

Opening Cue: Gently lifting and tucking your tailbone as you are lying down can release some muscle tension and increase circulation.

Cues: The suggestion is to practice Raising Your Heart 3 times.

1. When you are ready, put your feet on the floor under your knees.
2. As YOU breathe in, press down on your hips and shoulders, gently raising your heart as you arch your back a comfortable distance.
3. If you like, press your shoulders in toward your spine. Keep breathing in a comfortable way.
4. Notice your next breath in... On YOUR *next* long, slow breath out, slowly release, pull your legs in, and wrap your arms around your shins (or backs of your legs). Press as firmly as is comfortable for you today. If you like, we can practice another 2 Raising Your Heart flows. (**Repeat 2 more times.**)

B. BRIDGE LIFT AND RELEASE

Key Phrase: Long, slow breaths out *can* lower heart rate, lower blood pressure, and lower muscle tension.

Opening Cue: This bridge flow can strengthen core muscles.

Cues: When you are ready, put your feet on the floor under your knees again. The suggestion is to practice bridge lift and release 3 times.

1. As YOU breathe in, press down on your feet and gently lift your hips, any distance. (**Variation.**)
2. On YOUR next long, slow breath out, slowly release down and pull your knees in. Perhaps wrap your arms around your shins (or backs of your legs) and press as firmly as is comfortable. (**Repeat 3 times.**)
3. Still in a wrap, if you like, practice 3 comfortable breaths. As you breathe in, fingers press... As you breathe out, fingers release. (*Say 3 times slowly.*)

Variation: With your hips still lifted, extend your arms overhead, hands on the floor behind you. If you like, take 2 breaths here. Feel the breath in... Feel the breath out. (*Say 2 times slowly.*)

C. SIDE-TO-SIDE ROCKING

Key Phrase: Different days, different stretches.

Opening Cue: Gently moving can massage connective tissue, improve circulation, and reduce muscle tension.

Cues:

1. With your knees still pulled in, perhaps gently rock from side to side. If you like, wiggle your toes as you rock. Take your time as you rock.
2. Give yourself a moment to move your feet in any way that feels comfortable for you today. (**Variation.**)
3. When you are ready, notice your next breath in... Then on YOUR breath out, slowly release one leg to the floor.
4. Notice your next breath in... Then on YOUR breath out, slowly release the other leg to the floor.

Variation: Cross your ankles as you rock. When you are ready, reverse your ankles and continue rocking.

B. Seated
1. Get Yourself Set Up
Key Phrases: (1) Anything we do seated, you can do standing or even lying down. (2) You can always find ways to move and to breathe with me.

Opening Cue: Sitting or standing with your shoulders gently pressed back can take pressure off your back.

Cues:

1. Give yourself a few moments to find a comfortable way to sit today, either on a folded blanket or on a chair.
2. Gently press one shoulder back... Then press the other shoulder back.
3. If you like, move from side to side as you settle into your seat. Perhaps move in a circle. Take your time as you move. You may want to circle even more slowly the other way.
4. Make any adjustments to make your seat more comfortable.

2. Tip-to-Toe Stretch (photos on p.244)
Key Phrase: Different days, different stretches.

Opening Cue: We move slowly as we sit to practice "finding a better way to move."

Cues:

1. When you are ready, stretch one arm to the side or overhead, fingers stretched wide as you stretch from tip-to-toe.
2. Then stretch the other arm, either to the side or overhead, fingers stretched wide, gently lengthening the spine as you move.

3. Find your own rhythm as you stretch one arm and then the other.
4. Perhaps stretch your toes as you stretch your fingers. You also may like to lift your legs as you stretch. Take your time as you stretch from tip-to-toe.

3. Finger Stretch Breath

Key Phrase: Long, slow breaths out *can* lower heart rate, lower blood pressure, and lower muscle tension.

Opening Cue: You can interrupt your stress cycle by choosing how you breathe.

Cues: In Finger Stretch Breath, the suggestion is to stretch your fingers half an inch or a few centimeters. (**Variations.**)

1. When you are ready, gently press one shoulder back... Then press the other shoulder back.
2. If you like, let's practice 5 breaths. As YOU breathe in, fingers stretch... As YOU breathe out, release. (*Say 2 times slowly.*)
Always breathe in a comfortable way. On YOUR next breath in, fingers stretch... As YOU breathe out, release.
As YOU breathe in, fingers stretch... As YOU breathe out, release. (*Say 2 times slowly.*)
3. If you like, gently move the fingers on one hand or shake that hand... Then gently move the fingers on the other hand or shake that hand.

Variations: (1) Stretch just enough to notice the stretch. **Or** (2) Stretch your fingers as wide as you would like today. **Or** (3) Perhaps stretch your fingers in a different way today.

4. Neck and Shoulder Suite (a/b/c) (photos on p.255)

A. NECK MASSAGE

Key Phrase: Always move in a way that is comfortable for you today.

Opening Cue: Gently massaging muscles as you sit can reduce physical and emotional tension.

Cues:

1. The suggestion is to use one hand to massage the back of your neck, or if it's more comfortable for you today, the fronts of your shoulders. (**Variation.**)
2. Today you may want to: (*Slowly cue each as you move.*)
    a. Use one or both hands.

b. Gently tuck your chin and move your chin from side to side as you massage.
c. Massage the base of your neck/top of your back.
d. Gently lift and lower your chin as you massage.

Variation: Use a gentle or firm massage in a way that feels comfortable for you today.

B. CHIN LIFTS AND PENDULUM

Key Phrases: (1) You may be moving half an inch or a few centimeters, and that has benefits. (2) Some days, visualizing the stretch may be more helpful.

Opening Cue: The head weighs about 10 pounds or 5 kilograms. Gently stretching neck muscles can relieve some tension and pain.

Cues:

1. The suggestion is to practice this *slow* stretch 3 times. As YOU breathe in, chin slowly lifts... As YOU breathe out, chin slowly releases. (*Say slowly 3 times.*)
2. With your chin still released, slowly move your chin from side to side, like a pendulum. Take your time with each slow stretch.

C. NECK AND SHOULDER STRETCHES

Key Phrase: You can change how you are stretching any time; you are never stuck.

Opening Cue: Gently stretching muscles around the neck and shoulders as you sit can reduce some neck and back pain.

Cues:

1. We always do both sides. The suggestion is to gently release your *left* ear toward your *left* shoulder. Moving even half an inch or a few centimeters has benefit.
2. The suggestion is to move your *right* shoulder, doing each of these slow stretches 3 times:
    a. Press your shoulder forward... Then press it back. (*Say 3 times slowly.*)
    b. As YOU breathe in, lift that shoulder... As YOU breathe out, press that shoulder down as firmly as is comfortable for you today. If you like, hold this press for 2 more breaths. Hold the press...but not your breath. Feel the breath in... Feel the breath out. (*Say 2 times slowly.*) (**Repeat 2 more times.**)

    c. Now roll this shoulder forward 3 times in a comfortable way. Take your time with this slow stretch. When you are ready, roll this shoulder back 3 times. Again, take your time "to find a better way to move."
3. When you are ready, come back to sitting tall. If you like, let's do 2 sets of chin lifts. On YOUR breath in, chin slowly lifts… On YOUR breath out, chin slowly releases. (*Say 2 times slowly.*) (**Repeat #1–3 on the other side.**)

5. Shoulder Rock 'n Roll (photo on p.254)

Key Phrase: Different days, different stretches.

Opening Cue: Gentle shoulder stretches as you sit can reduce some neck and back pain.

Cues:

1. Gently bend your elbows and stretch your fingers if that is comfortable for you today.
2. When you are ready, move one arm across the front, the other arm across the back as we practice shoulder Rock 'n Roll. Leading from the elbows if you like, now move the other arm across the front, and the other across the back. That's 1 set. Find your own rhythm as you practice 2 more sets. You can make each stretch as gentle or intense as you need today. Moving the arms from front to back in any way that feels comfortable… Finding your own rhythm as you move.
3. Now if you like, lead from the shoulders as you move from front to back. Practice as many sets as feels comfortable for you today… Moving the arms from front to back as slowly as you would like.
4. Now, the suggestion is to hold the stretch on each side for 2 breaths. As one shoulder moves across the front and the other across the back, hold the stretch…but not your breath. Feel the breath in… Feel the breath out. (*Say 2 times slowly.*)
5. Now as your other shoulder moves across the front and the other across the back, hold the stretch…but not your breath. Feel the breath in… Feel the breath out. (*Say 2 times slowly.*)
6. When you are ready, arms to your sides.

6. Shoulder Rolls (photos on p.254)

Key Phrase: Today you may want to practice long breaths out.

Opening Cue: Long, slow breaths out can reduce muscle tension.

Cues:

1. When you are ready, let's practice 3 shoulder rolls forward and 3 shoulder rolls back. As YOU breathe in, shoulders lift... As YOU breathe out, shoulders roll forward and down. (*Say 3 times slowly.*)
   Always move in a comfortable way.
2. Now 3 back. As YOU breathe in, shoulders lift... As YOU breathe out, shoulders roll back and down. (*Say 3 times slowly.*)

Variations: (1) After one roll: if you like, move even more slowly on the next two rolls. **Or** (2) After two rolls: if you like, stop halfway down the next roll. Hold the stretch...but not your breath.

7. Feel the Breath
Key Phrase: Longer breaths in *can* be energizing.

Opening Cue: Noticing your breath can be the first step in managing how you breathe.

Cues:

1. When you are ready, gently press one shoulder back... Then press the other shoulder back.
2. If you like, put one or both hands over your heart... Put one or both hands over your heart.
3. The suggestion is to take 3 breaths. Today you may want to practice longer breaths in.
   Feel the breath in... Feel the breath out. (*Say 3 times slowly.*)
4. If you like, gently move the fingers on one hand or shake that hand... Then gently move the fingers on the other hand or shake that hand.

8. Physiological Sigh
Key Phrase: Practicing the physiological sigh 2 or 3 times can help lower carbon dioxide levels in the blood, which can lower anxiety.

Opening Cue: You can interrupt your stress cycle by choosing how you breathe.

Cues:

1. When you are ready, gently press one shoulder back... Then press the other shoulder back.
2. Let's practice once. Always move and breathe in a comfortable way.
   When you are ready, practice a deep breath in and stretch your fingers

wide. Then breathe in more...perhaps stretch your fingers a little more. Hold that breath as long as you like...when you are ready, SIGH it out, fingers release. The suggestion is to practice 2 more times. (*Say 2 more times slowly.*)

3. If you like, gently move the fingers on one hand or shake that hand... Then gently move the fingers on the other hand or shake that hand.
4. The physiological sigh is a way to practice lowering your anxiety levels in 2 or 3 breaths.

C. Make a Plan

Opening Cue: Next time you start to feel pain or discomfort, you can have a 1- to 2-minute plan ready to go.

Cues:

1. The suggestion is to choose one breath we did today. We did Feel the Breath, Finger Stretch Breath, and the physiological sigh. Long, slow breaths out *can* lower blood pressure. So now you have a 1-minute breath to do later when you want to change how you are feeling.
2. If you like, add one stretch to do again. Perhaps include 1-2-3 Shoulder Stretch or shoulder Rock 'n Roll. You now have a 2-minute plan to manage your pain.
3. (See www.greentreeyoga.org/pain-management-resources for free downloads.)

D. Extras

1. Time Adjustments

Running Out of Time? When you notice you are running out of time, move ahead to the physiological sigh. Then Make a Plan.

Too Much Time? After the physiological sigh, repeat seated shoulder Rock 'n Roll, shoulder rolls, and Finger Stretch Breath.

2. Theme Variation: The Pause (Take 2)

After you have done this practice several times, you can offer this idea at the beginning and mention it a few times during the practice:

> Today, you might want to notice if you pause between the breath in and the breath out. You don't need to change it, unless you want to play with pausing and noticing it.

VII. REST AND RESTORE 1 (LYING DOWN)

Note: Before you teach, please review In Case You Missed It... (p.101)

A. Lying Down
1. Get Yourself Set Up (photos on p.258)
Key Phrases: (1) Anything we do lying down, you can do seated or standing. (2) You can always find ways to move and to breathe with me.

Opening Cue: Major muscles that usually work to hold us up can release when we lie down.

Cues: Give yourself a few moments to get yourself set up. You can make adjustments; you are never stuck.

1. As you sit on the floor, you may want a rolled-up blanket, towel, or mat under your knees before you lie back.
2. One suggestion is to place a rolled-up mat or blanket along your spine with support for your head.

2. Feel the Breath
Key Phrase: Long, slow breaths out *can* lower heart rate, lower blood pressure, and lower muscle tension.

Opening Cue: One way we can manage pain in real-time is by choosing how we breathe.

Cues:

1. When you are ready, gently press one shoulder back... Then press the other shoulder back.
2. If you like, put one or both hands over your heart... Put one or both hands over your heart.
3. The suggestion is to practice 5 breaths. Today you may like to practice long, slow breaths out.
   Feel the breath in... Feel the breath out. (*Say 2 times slowly.*)
   Always breathe in a comfortable way.
   Feel the breath in... Feel the breath out. (*Say 3 times slowly.*)
4. If you like, gently move the fingers on one hand or shake that hand... Then gently move the fingers on the other hand or shake that hand.

Variation: If you like, after you feel the breath in, pause long enough to notice the pause, then feel the breath out.

3. Tip-to-Toe Stretch (photos on p.258)

Key Phrase: Always move in a comfortable way.

Opening Cue: Lying down allows different sets of large muscles to release.

Cues:

1. When you are ready, stretch one arm to the side or overhead as we stretch from tip-to-toe. Then stretch the other arm. Perhaps stretch your fingers wide.
2. The suggestion is to find your own rhythm as you move in any way that is comfortable for you today. Take your time with the stretch.
3. When you are ready, press one heel forward and then the other. Keep stretching your arms and pressing the heels forward in any way that feels comfortable for you today. Notice where you feel the stretch as you slowly move.
4. If you like, stretch your fingers and your toes 3 times. As YOU breathe in, stretch… As YOU breathe out, release. (*Say 3 times slowly.*)
5. When you are ready, arms by your sides.

4. Bridge Flow (a/b) (photos on p.259)

A. RAISING YOUR HEART

Key Phrase: Use the pieces of the stretch that feel comfortable for you today.

Opening Cue: Gently lifting and tucking your tailbone as you are lying down can release some muscle tension and increase circulation.

Cues: The suggestion is to practice Raising Your Heart 3 times.

1. When you are ready, put your feet on the floor under your knees.
2. As YOU breathe in, press down on your hips and shoulders, gently raising your heart as you arch your back a comfortable distance.
3. If you like, press your shoulders in toward your spine. Keep breathing in a comfortable way.
4. Notice your next breath in… On YOUR *next* long, slow breath out, slowly release, pull your legs in, and wrap your arms around your shins (or backs of your legs). Press as firmly as is comfortable for you today. If you like, we can practice another 2 Raising Your Heart flows. (**Repeat 2 more times.**)

B. BRIDGE LIFT AND RELEASE

Key Phrase: Long, slow breaths out *can* lower heart rate, lower blood pressure, and lower muscle tension.

Opening Cue: This bridge flow can strengthen core muscles.

Cues: When you are ready, put your feet on the floor under your knees again. The suggestion is to practice bridge lift and release 3 times.

1. As YOU breathe in, press down on your feet and gently lift your hips, any distance. (**Variation.**)
2. On YOUR next long, slow breath out, slowly release down and pull your knees in. Perhaps wrap your arms around your shins or backs of your legs and press as firmly as is comfortable. (**Repeat 3 times.**)
3. Still in a wrap, if you like, practice 3 comfortable breaths. As you breathe in, fingers press... As you breathe out, fingers release. (*Say 3 times slowly.*)

Variation: With your hips still lifted, extend your arms overhead, hands on the floor behind you. If you like, take 2 breaths here. Feel the breath in... Feel the breath out. (*Say 2 times slowly.*)

5. Hip-to-Toe Stretches (a/b/c/d/e/f) (photos on p.261)

A. TOES, FOOT, AND ANKLE 1

Key Phrase: Small movements have benefits—even half an inch or a few centimeters.

Opening Cue: Gentle stretches can take pressure off joints and improve circulation.

Cues:

1. We always do both sides. When you are ready, rest one leg on the floor and bend your other knee.
2. Wrap your hands around the front of your shin or the back of your leg.
3. The suggestion is to slowly move that foot in a circle. When you are ready, slowly circle the other way.
4. If you like, stretch all your toes on both feet 3 times. On YOUR breath in, stretch your toes... As YOU breathe out, release. (*Say 3 times slowly.*)

B. TOES, FOOT, AND ANKLE 2

Key Phrase: Put as much muscle energy into the stretch as feels comfortable for you today.

Opening Cue: We move slowly to practice "finding a better way to move."

Cues:

1. When you are ready, move that foot 3 times, as if pressing a gas pedal.

Slowly press the toes away and then pull the toes toward your shin. Now if you like, hold each stretch for 2 breaths. Hold the stretch...but not the breath. Press your toes away. Feel the breath in... Feel the breath out. (*Say 2 times slowly.*) Then pull the toes toward you. Feel the breath in... Feel the breath out. (*Say 2 times slowly.*) (**Variations.**)

2. If you like, stretch all your toes 3 times again. As YOU breathe in, stretch your toes... As YOU breathe out, release. (*Say 3 times slowly.*)

Variations: (1) If you like, move that foot 3 times from side to side, like a windshield wiper. **Or** (2) If you like, slowly circle that foot in a comfortable way. When you are ready, circle the other way.

C. KNEE STRETCH

Key Phrase: Always move in a way that is comfortable for you today.

Opening Cue: Small, gentle stretches can keep the knee joints healthy and lubricated, which can reduce pain.

Cues:

1. Hold the top part of your leg (femur) steady as you circle the foot, as if drawing on the wall in front of you. (**Variation.**) The gentle movement can massage tendons and ligaments as well as lengthen muscles. It can be any size circle or any shape that is comfortable for you today.
2. When you are ready, slowly move in the other direction.

Variation: If you feel like being silly today, imagine drawing with a color crayon that makes you feel silly.

D. SPIRAL HIP STRETCH

Key Phrase: Different days, different stretches.

Opening Cue: Moving slowly allows you to gently stretch hip muscles and lubricate the hip joints.

Cues:

1. When you are ready, release your hands to your sides, knee still bent as we do the spiral hip stretch. Begin to move that knee in a circle or shape that feels comfortable.
2. Perhaps today sweep that leg across to the other side and then pull it toward you making a different spiral. Take your time with these stretches to lubricate the hip joint. When you are ready, circle the other way.

E. OUTER HIP STRETCH/TWIST

Key Phrase: There is no place you are trying to go with a stretch.

Opening Cue: Let's gently stretch the outer hip muscles and the spine.

Cues:

1. When you are ready, place your foot above or next to the knee on the other leg. Gently draw that knee across. Even small movements have benefits.
2. If you like, look the opposite way for a full spinal twist. Stay here for 4 more breaths if that is comfortable for you today. Feel the breath in… Feel the breath out. (*Say 4 times slowly.*)

Variation: For these 4 breaths: As YOU breathe in, fingers press. As YOU breathe out, release the press.

F. BACK RELEASE 1

Key Phrase: Use the pieces of the stretch that feel comfortable for you today.

Opening Cue: The suggestion is to take long, slow breaths out if that is comfortable for you today.

Cues: When you are ready, put both feet on the floor under your knees. Let's practice this back release 3 times.

1. As YOU breathe in, press down on your feet and gently lift your hips, any distance…
   As YOU breathe out, slowly release down, and on the same long, slow breath out, pull your knees in and wrap your arms around your shins (or backs of your legs). (*Say 3 times slowly.*)
2. Now, with your arms still around your legs, let's practice 3 breaths. As YOU breathe in, fingers press… As YOU breathe out, fingers release. (*Say 3 times slowly.*)
3. Notice your next breath in… As YOU breathe out, slowly release one leg to the floor. Notice your next breath in… As YOU breathe out, slowly release the other leg to the floor. (**Repeat a/b/c/d/e/f on the other side.**)

6. Feel the Breath with Fingertip Press

Key Phrases: (1) Longer breaths in *can* be energizing. (2) Long, slow breaths out *can* lower blood pressure. (*Or choose one of these phrases based on what fits the needs of the class.*)

Opening Cue: Noticing your breath can be a first step in managing how you breathe.

Cues:

1. When you are ready, gently press one shoulder back... Then press the other shoulder back.
2. If you like, put one or both hands over your heart... Put one or both hands over your heart.
3. Let's practice 5 breaths. Feel the breath in, fingertips press... Feel the breath out, release the press. (*Say 2 times slowly.*)
   Always breathe in a comfortable way.
   Feel the breath in, fingertips press... Feel the breath out, release. (*Say 3 times slowly.*)
4. If you like, gently move the fingers on one hand or shake that hand... Then gently move the fingers on the other hand or shake that hand.

7. 1-2-3 Shoulder Stretches (a/b/c)

A. 1-2-3 SINGLE SHOULDER STRETCH

Key Phrase: We move slowly so you can "find a better way to move."

Opening Cue: Gently stretching muscles around the neck and shoulders as you lie down can reduce muscle and emotional tension.

Cues:

1. Let's practice 3 sets of 1-2-3 single shoulder stretch. We always do both sides.
2. As YOU breathe in, lift one shoulder up... That's 1. As YOU breathe out, press that same shoulder down... That's 2. Then release the press... That's 3. And that's 1 set of 1-2-3 shoulder stretch. (*Say 3 times slowly.*)
3. Now let's practice the stretch on the other shoulder. (**Repeat on the other side.**)

B. 1-2-3 DOUBLE SHOULDER STRETCH

Key Phrase: Make each stretch as gentle or intense as you need today.

Opening Cue: You can continue to release emotional and physical tension as you are lying down.

Cues:

1. Let's practice 3 sets of 1-2-3 double shoulder stretch.
2. As YOU breathe in, lift both shoulders up... That's 1. As YOU breathe out,

press both shoulders down... That's 2. Then release the press... That's 3. And that's 1 set. The suggestion is to practice 2 more sets. (*Say 3 times slowly.*)

C. 1-2-3 SIDE-TO-SIDE SHOULDER STRETCH
Key Phrase: Always move in a comfortable way.

Opening Cue: Gently releasing muscle tension as you are lying down can have many benefits.

Cues:

1. If you like, you can practice 3 sets of 1-2-3 side-to-side shoulder stretch with your arms by your sides.
2. As YOU breathe in, lift one shoulder toward your ear and press the other shoulder away from the other ear... That's 1. As YOU breathe out, lift the other shoulder toward your ear and press the other shoulder away from the other ear... That's 2. Then release both shoulders... That's 3. And that's 1 set. The suggestion is to practice 2 more sets. (*Say 3 times slowly.*)

Variation: When you are ready, arc one arm overhead in a comfortable way, if you like, fingers stretched wide. Then the other arm overhead, fingers stretched wide.

8. Back Release 2: Knee Circles (photos on p.260)
Key Phrase: We move slowly so you can "find a better way to move."

Opening Cue: Gently moving as you are lying down can massage connective tissue and reduce muscle tension.

Cues:

1. When you are ready, place your hands by your sides with your palms down and your feet under your knees. If it is more comfortable, keep your feet on the floor. A different stretch is to lift both knees.
2. The suggestion is to move your knees in a circle, a spiral, or any comfortable shape. (**Variation.**) Take your time with the gentle stretch to massage the low back. When you are ready, move in the other direction. Move slowly as you "find a better way to move."
3. When you are ready, pull both knees toward you again and wrap your arms around your shins or backs of your legs. Give yourself a moment here to press as firmly as is comfortable. If you like, take 2 breaths. Feel the breath in... Feel the breath out. (*Say 2 times slowly.*) When you are

ready, notice your next breath in... As YOU breathe out, release one leg to the floor. Notice your next breath in... As YOU breathe out, release the other leg to the floor.

Variation: For a moment of silliness, imagine colorful crayons on your knees as you draw on the ceiling. Perhaps choose a color that makes you feel... (silly, cheerful, playful...)

9. Tip-to-Toe Stretch (Repeat #3)

10. Anytime, Anywhere Breath
Key Phrase: A long, slow breath out can lower heart rate, lower blood pressure, and lower muscle tension.

Opening Cue: Noticing your breath can be the first step in managing how you breathe.

Cues: You can do the Anytime, Anywhere Breath even when talking with someone.

1. When you are ready, gently press one shoulder back... Then press the other shoulder back. If you like, place one hand on your leg in a way that is comfortable for you today.
2. Let's practice 5 breaths. The suggestion is to take long, slow breaths out. (**Variation 1.**)
   As YOU breathe in, fingers press... As YOU breathe out, release. (*Say 2 times slowly.*)
   Always breathe in a comfortable way.
   On YOUR next breath in, fingers press... As YOU breathe out, release. As YOU breathe in, fingers press... As YOU breathe out, release. (*Say 2 times slowly.*)
3. If you like, gently move the fingers on one hand or shake that hand... Then gently move the fingers on the other hand or shake that hand. (**Variation 2.**)
4. You may want to practice the Anytime, Anywhere Breath later, when you want to change how you are feeling.

Variations: (1) Press your fingers firmly or gently today. **Or** (2) Now if you like, use your other hand and practice saying it 3 times to yourself in your mind, since *you* are always with you. (*Say slowly during this time so there is no "dead air." Don't rush your words... Don't rush your breath. Take your time with your words... Take your time with your breath.*)

B. Make a Plan
Opening Cue: Next time you start to feel pain or discomfort, you can have a 1- to 2-minute plan ready to go.

Cues:

1. The suggestion is to choose one breath we did today. We did Feel the Breath, Feel the Breath with fingertip press, and the Anytime, Anywhere Breath. Long, slow breaths out *can* lower blood pressure. So now you have a 1-minute breath to do later when you want to change how you are feeling.
2. If you like, add one stretch to do again. Perhaps include 1-2-3 Shoulder Stretches or the Tip-to-Toe Stretch. You now have a 2-minute plan to manage your pain.
3. (See www.greentreeyoga.org/pain-management-resources for free downloads.)

C. Extras
1. Time Adjustments
Running Out of Time? When you notice you are running out of time, move ahead to the Anytime, Anywhere Breath and Make a Plan.

Too Much Time? After the Anytime, Anywhere Breath, repeat the bridge flow: Raising Your Heart and bridge lift and release.

2. Theme Variation: Savor the Stretch
After you have done this practice several times, you can offer this idea at the beginning and mention it a few times during the practice:

> Today, you might want to move even more slowly than in our last practice. Give yourself a moment to Savor the Stretch.

VIII. REST AND RESTORE 2 (STANDING/ SEATED/LYING DOWN)
Note: Please read In Case You Missed It... (p.101)

A. Standing
1. Tip-to-Toe Stretch (photos on p.243)
Key Phrase: As Moshé Feldenkrais said, "There isn't a right way to move; there is a better way to move."

Opening Cue: We start standing to gently stretch from tip-to-toe before we take a seat.

Cues:

1. When you are ready, stretch one arm to the side or overhead, fingers stretched wide in the Tip-to-Toe Stretch.
2. Then stretch the other arm, either to the side or overhead, fingers stretched wide.
3. The suggestion is to find your own rhythm as you stretch one arm and then the other. We move slowly so you can "find a better way to move" toward a healthier spine.
4. When you are ready, put your hands on your hips.
5. If you like, lift one heel and press on your toes. Then lift the other heel and press on the toes. Let's practice that two more times. (*Say 2 times slowly.*)

2. Wide-Legged Add-On (photos on p.245)

Key Phrase: Even moving half an inch or a few centimeters has benefits; it means muscles are not getting tighter.

Opening Cue: Another way we can manage pain is with gentle stretches to reduce pressure on nerves and joints.

Cues:

1. When you are ready, step your feet apart, hands on your hips as we do the wide-legged add-on. (**Variation.**)
2. In whatever way feels comfortable, move one hip to one side… Then move the other hip to the other side. We move slowly so you can "find a better way to move."
3. Today you may like to add lifting your shoulder in a gentle arc as you move to one side… Then lift the other shoulder in a gentle arc as you move the other hip to the side. Find your own rhythm as you move from side to side. Take your time as you move.
4. When you are ready, come back to standing tall. If you like, gently *stretch* the fingers on one hand or shake that hand… Then gently *stretch* the fingers or shake the other hand.

Variation: If you like, roll from the inside edges to the outside edges of your feet… Roll from the inside to the outside edges of your feet in a comfortable way.

B. Seated
1. Get Yourself Set Up
Key Phrase: Always move in a comfortable way.

Opening Cue: Sitting or standing with your shoulders gently pressed back can take pressure off your back.

Cues:

1. Give yourself a few moments to find a comfortable way to sit today, either on a folded blanket or on a chair.
2. Gently press one shoulder back, and then press the other shoulder back.
3. If you like, move from side to side as you settle into your seat. Perhaps move in a circle. Take your time as you move. You may want to circle even more slowly the other way.
4. Make any adjustments to find your seat more comfortable.

2. Feel the Breath
Key Phrase: Long, slow breaths out *can* lower heart rate, lower blood pressure, and lower muscle tension.

Opening Cue: One way we can manage pain in real-time is by choosing how we breathe.

Cues:

1. When you are ready, gently press one shoulder back... Then press the other shoulder back.
2. If you like, put one or both hands over your heart... Put one or both hands over your heart.
3. The suggestion is to take 5 breaths. Today you may like to practice long breaths out.
   Feel the breath in... Feel the breath out. (*Say 2 times slowly.*)
   Always breathe in a comfortable way.
   Feel the breath in... Feel the breath out. (*Say 3 times slowly.*)
4. If you like, gently move the fingers on one hand or shake that hand... Then gently move the fingers on the other hand or shake that hand.

3. Cat/Cow (photos on p.242)
Key Phrase: Different days, different stretches.

Opening Cue: Bending forward and back (flexing and extending) the spine as you sit are two more ways you can move toward a healthier spine.

Cues:

1. If you like, tap your *fingertips* on your legs. The suggestion is to practice seated cat/cow 2 times.
2. As YOU breathe in, chin lifts...shoulders back...rock forward.
   As YOU breathe out, chin tucks...shoulders forward...rock back a comfortable distance. Always move and breathe in a comfortable way.
3. On YOUR next breath in, chin lifts...shoulders back...rock forward. As YOU breathe out, chin tucks...shoulders forward...rock back a comfortable distance.
4. When you are ready, come back to sitting tall.

4. Shoulder Rolls (photos on p.254)

Key Phrase: Today you may want to practice long breaths out.

Opening Cue: Long breaths out *can* reduce muscle tension.

Cues:

1. The suggestion is to practice 3 shoulder rolls forward and 3 shoulder rolls back. As YOU breathe in, shoulders lift... As YOU breathe out, shoulders roll forward and down. (*Say 3 times slowly.*)
   Always move in a comfortable way.
2. Now 3 back. As YOU breathe in, shoulders lift... As YOU breathe out, shoulders roll back and down. (*Say 3 times slowly.*)

C. Lying Down
1. Get Yourself Set Up (p. 218)
2. Final Stretch: A Body-Based, Guided Meditation
(15 minutes): Either version #1 or #2 (see p.218)

D. Seated
1. Get Yourself Set Up

1. Give yourself a few moments to find a comfortable seat.
2. Gently press one shoulder back, and then press the other shoulder back.
3. If you like, move from side to side as you settle into your seat.

2. 1-2-3 Shoulder Stretch (photos on p.254)

Key Phrases: (1) Even small stretches have benefits. (2) Long, slow breaths out *can* lower blood pressure.

Opening Cue: The suggestion is to practice 1-2-3 Shoulder Stretch 3 times.

Cues:

1. Gently bend your elbows with fingers stretched wide if that is comfortable for you today.
2. As YOU breathe in, shoulders and elbows press back... That's 1.
   As YOU breathe out, shoulders and elbows press forward... That's 2.
   And release... That's 3. And that's 1 set. You can make each stretch as gentle or intense as you need today.
3. The suggestion is to practice 2 more sets of 1-2-3 Shoulder Stretch. (*Say slowly 2 more times.*)

3. Finger Stretch Breath

Key Phrase: Long, slow breaths out *can* lower heart rate, lower blood pressure, and lower muscle tension.

Opening Cue: You can interrupt your stress cycle by choosing how you breathe.

Cues: In Finger Stretch Breath, the suggestion is to stretch your fingers half an inch or a few centimeters. (**Variations.**)

1. When you are ready, gently press one shoulder back... Then press the other shoulder back. If you like, let's practice 5 breaths.
2. As YOU breathe in, fingers stretch... As YOU breathe out, release. (*Say 2 times slowly.*)
   Always breathe in a comfortable way.
   On YOUR next breath in, fingers stretch... As YOU breathe out, release.
   As YOU breathe in, fingers stretch... As YOU breathe out, release. (*Say 2 times slowly.*)
3. If you like, gently move the fingers on one hand or shake that hand... Then gently move the fingers on the other hand or shake that hand.

Variations: (1) Stretch just enough to notice the stretch. **Or** (2) Stretch your fingers as wide as you would like today. **Or** (3) Perhaps stretch your fingers in a different way today.

E. Make a Plan

Opening Cue: Next time you start to feel pain or discomfort, you can have a 1- to 2-minute plan ready to go.

Cues:

1. The suggestion is to choose one breath we did today. We did Feel the Breath and Finger Stretch Breath. A long breath out *can* lower blood

pressure. So now you have a 1-minute breath to do later when you want to change how you are feeling.
2. If you like, add one stretch you might like to do again. Perhaps include 1-2-3 Shoulder Stretch or Tip-to-Toe Stretch. You now have a 2-minute plan to manage your pain.
3. (See www.greentreeyoga.org/pain-management-resources for free downloads.)

F. Extras
1. Time Adjustments
Running Out of Time? Move from Final Stretch to Make a Plan.

Too Much Time? Include cat/cow and shoulder rolls from B. Seated.

2. Theme Variation: Savor the Stretch
After you have done this practice several times, you can offer this idea at the beginning and mention it a few times during the practice:

> Today, you might want to move even more slowly than in our last practice. Give yourself a moment to Savor the Stretch.

CHAPTER 8

Sixty- to Ninety-Minute Practices

Outlines and Practice Sequences

*Note: * Add for a 90-minute practice.*

I. Building Strength (Standing/Seated/Lying Down)
A. Standing (20 minutes)

1. Tip-to-Toe Stretch with Balance
2. Wide-Legged Add-On
3. Feel the Breath
4. Hip Stretch and Core Strengthening Flow: a. Pendulum and Pedal the Feet; * *Hip and Core Flow*; * *Finger Stretch Breath*; b. Tree Pose; * *Tree Pose #4*
5. Feel the Breath with Fingertip Press
6. Warrior 1 Flow: a. Achilles Tendon and Calf Stretch; b. Warrior 1; c. Warrior 1 with a Twist; d. Tip-to-Toe Stretch; e. Anytime, Anywhere Breath; * *Eagle Flow (p.151)*

B. Seated (10 minutes)

1. Get Yourself Set Up
2. Physiological Sigh
3. Shoulder Rolls
4. Core Check: * *Find a New Stretch (p.114)*; * *1-2-3 Shoulder Stretch*
5. Feel the Breath with Fingertip Press

C. Lying Down (15 minutes)

1. Get Yourself Set Up
2. The Noticing Breath
3. Gentle Twist with Knees: * *The Noticing Breath (p.110)*
4. Bridge Flow: a. Raising Your Heart; b. Bridge Lift and Release; c. Side-to-Side Rocking; * *Repeat a stretch*

D. Final Stretch (15 minutes)

1. Get Yourself Set Up: * *The Noticing Breath*
2. Final Stretch: A Body-Based, Guided Meditation

E. Make a Plan: Practice the breath and movement

F. Extras

1. Time Adjustments
2. Theme Variation: Little Changes
3. Ideas to extend to a 90-minute practice: Seated; Lying Down

II. Stretch, Breathe, Rest, and Restore (Standing/Seated/Lying Down)
A. Standing (5 minutes)

1. Tip-to-Toe Stretch
2. Wide-Legged Add-On
3. Feel the Breath

B. Seated (15 minutes)

1. Get Yourself Set Up
2. The Wave Breath
3. Neck and Shoulder Suite: a. Neck Massage; b. Chin Lifts and Pendulum; c. Neck and Shoulder Stretches
4. Shoulder Rolls
5. Finger Stretch Breath: * *Shoulder Suite (p.126)*
6. Classic Twist with Cat/Cow

C. Lying Down (25 minutes)

1. Get Yourself Set Up
2. The Noticing Breath: * *Tip-to-Toe Stretch*; * *Crescent Stretch*; * *Shoulder Stretches*
3. Bridge Flow: a. Raising Your Heart; b. Bridge Lift and Release; c. Side-to-Side Rocking
4. Gentle Twist with Knees: * *Side-to-Side Rocking*; * *#4 Stretch Flow*
5. Feel the Breath with Fingertip Press
6. Hip-to-Toe Stretches: a. Toes, Foot, and Ankle 1; b. Toes, Foot, and Ankle 2; c. Knee Stretch; d. Spiral Hip Stretch; e. Outer Hip Stretch/Twist; f. Back Release 1

D. Final Stretch (15 minutes)

1. Get Yourself Set Up: * *The Noticing Breath (p.110)*
2. Final Stretch: A Body-Based, Guided Meditation

E. Make a Plan: * **Practice the breath and movement**

F. Extras

1. Time Adjustments
2. Theme Variation: Savor the Stretch
3. Ideas to extend to a 90-minute practice: Seated; Lying Down; Final Stretch

III: Gently Moving Toward a Healthier Spine (Standing/Seated/Lying Down)
A. Standing (15 minutes)

1. Tip-to-Toe Stretch
2. Feel the Breath
3. Side-to-Side (lateral) Stretches: a. Crescent Stretch; b. Wide-Legged Add-On
4. Kitchen Stretch: a. Setup; b. Strong and Steady; c. Hip Rock 'n Roll; * *Gentle Backbend*
5. Twists: a. Gentle Twist: Standing Behind Chair; b. Gentle Twist: Foot on Chair Seat
6. Tip-to-Toe Stretch

B. Seated (15 minutes)

1. Get Yourself Set Up
2. The Wave Breath
3. Tip-to-Toe Stretch
4. Side-to-Side (lateral) Stretches: a. Shoulder Lift and Release; b. Crescent Stretch
5. Cat/Cow (Flex and Extend): * *Shoulder Suite (p.126)*
6. Twists and Cat/Cow: a. Shoulder Rock 'n Roll; b. Classic Twist with Cat/Cow
7. Finger Stretch Breath

C. Lying Down (15 minutes)

1. Get Yourself Set Up
2. The Noticing Breath
3. Tip-to-Toe Stretch
4. Side-to-Side (lateral) Stretches: Shoulder Lift and Release; * *Crescent Stretch*; * *Feel the Breath with Fingertip Press*
5. Bridge Flow: a. Raising Your Heart; b. Bridge Lift and Release
6. Twists: a. Outer Hip Stretch/Twist; b. Side-to-Side Rocking; * *#4 with Variation*
7. Anytime, Anywhere Breath

D. Final Stretch (15 minutes) (see p.218)

1. Get Yourself Set Up: * *The Noticing Breath (p.110)*
2. Final Stretch: A Body-Based, Guided Meditation

E. Make a Plan: * Practice the breath and movement

F. Extras

1. Time Adjustments
2. Theme Variation: Savor the Stretch
3. Ideas to extend to a 90-minute practice: Supported Backbend; Crescent Stretch Variation; 1-2-3 Shoulder Stretch Variation; Extended Make a Plan

PRACTICE SEQUENCES

I. BUILDING STRENGTH (STANDING/SEATED/LYING DOWN)
Note: Before you teach, please review In Case You Missed It... (p.101)

A. Standing (20 minutes)
1. Tip-to-Toe Stretch with Balance (photo on p.243)
Key Phrase: When we do not move, tight muscles can press on nerves and joints.

Opening Cue: As Moshé Feldenkrais said, "There isn't a right way to move; there is a better way to move."

Cues:

1. When you are ready, stretch one arm to the side or overhead, fingers stretched wide in the Tip-to-Toe Stretch.
2. Then stretch the other arm, either to the side or overhead, fingers stretched wide, gently lengthening the spine as you move.
3. Find your own rhythm as you stretch one arm and then the other. We move slowly so you can "find a better way to move."
4. If you like, as you arc one arm overhead, lift that foot to the side any distance. You are building strength as you find your balance. Then stretch to the other side and lift that leg out to the side. When you are ready, come back to standing tall with your hands on your hips.
5. If you like, lift one heel and press on the toes. Then lift the other heel and press on the toes. The suggestion is to practice the toe stretch 2 more times. (*Say 2 times slowly.*)

2. Wide-Legged Add-On (photos on p.245)
Key Phrase: Moving even half an inch or a few centimeters has benefits; it means muscles are not getting tighter.

Opening Cue: Another way we can manage pain is with gentle stretches to reduce pressure on nerves and lubricate joints.

Cues:

1. When you are ready, step your feet apart, hands on your hips as we do the wide-legged add-on. (**Variation.**)
2. In whatever way feels comfortable, move one hip to one side... Then move the other hip to the other side. We move slowly so you can "find a better way to move."

3. Today you may like to add lifting your shoulder in a gentle arc as you move to one side... Then lift the other shoulder in a gentle arc as you move the other hip to the side. Find your own rhythm as you move from side to side. Take your time as you move.
4. When you are ready, come back to standing tall. If you like, gently *stretch* the fingers on one hand or shake that hand... Then gently *stretch* the fingers or shake the other hand.

Variation: Today you may want to roll from the inside edges to the outside edges of your feet... Roll from the inside to the outside edges in any way that is comfortable for you today.

3. Feel the Breath
Key Phrase: Long, slow breaths out *can* lower heart rate, lower blood pressure, and lower muscle tension.

Opening Cue: You can interrupt your stress cycle by choosing how you breathe.

Cues:

1. When you are ready, gently press one shoulder back... Then press the other shoulder back.
2. If you like, put one or both hands over your heart... Put one or both hands over your heart.
3. Let's practice 5 breaths. Today you may like to practice long breaths out. Feel the breath in... Feel the breath out. (*Say 2 times slowly.*) Always breathe in a comfortable way. Feel the breath in... Feel the breath out. (*Say 3 times slowly.*)
4. If you like, gently move the fingers on one hand or shake that hand... Then gently move the fingers on the other hand or shake that hand.

Variations: (1) If you like, after you feel the breath in, pause long enough to notice the pause, then... Feel the breath out... **Or** (2) If you like, after you feel the breath out, pause long enough to notice the pause, then feel the breath in...

4. Hip Stretch and Core Strengthening Flow (a/b) (photos on p.253)
A. PENDULUM AND PEDAL THE FEET
Key Phrase: Different day, different stretches.

Opening Cue: Another way to manage pain is to strengthen muscles, especially the core muscles that wrap around the front and back.

Cues: A slight bend in your standing leg can protect the knee joint.

1. We always do both sides. The suggestion is to slowly move your leg from side to side like a pendulum.
2. You may want to take your hand off the chair. You build core muscles as you move to find your balance. When your hand is on the chair, you can focus on the stretch. (**Variation.**)
3. When you are ready, put your foot down and your hands on your hips.
4. Give yourself a moment to lift one heel, press on the toes. Then lift the other heel, press on the toes. If you like, practice 2 more sets, making the press as firm or as gentle as you need today.

Variation: If you like, move your leg in a circle, a spiral, or in any comfortable way. Then, perhaps move it even more slowly as you move in the other direction.

B. TREE POSE (PHOTOS ON P.240)

Key Phrase: You can move your foot anytime; you are never stuck.

Opening Cue: We can strengthen core muscles as we find our balance in tree pose.

Cues: We always do both sides. The suggestion is to turn your knee open and find a place to press your foot that makes you feel strong today. But pressing your foot on your knee can put pressure on that joint. Today, you may want your hand on the chair to focus on the stretch. When you take it off the chair, notice how you move to find your balance and build core muscles.

1. (*Side 1.*) Let's practice 3 breaths. You may want to practice long, slow breaths out today.
   As YOU breathe in, one or both arms open, fingers stretched wide... As YOU breathe out, hands over your heart. (*Say 3 times slowly.*) When you're ready, come back to standing tall or... (**Variation.**)
2. Give yourself a moment to lift one heel, press on the toes. Then lift the other heel, press on the toes. If you like, practice 2 more sets, making the press as firm or as gentle as you need today.
3. (*Side 2.*) (**Repeat on the other side.**) If you like, lift one or both arms to the side or overhead. Let's practice 3 breaths.
   As YOU breathe in, fingers spread wide... As YOU breathe out, fingers release. (*Say 3 times slowly.*)
4. Perhaps move your arms and notice as you find your balance. When you are ready, come back to standing tall or... (**Variation.**)

Variation (both sides): Today you may want to take up space to come out of tree pose. On YOUR breath in, extend your leg to the side, stretching your arms and fingers wide. You may want to hold the stretch…but not your breath. When you notice you are breathing…when you notice you are breathing, wiggle your fingers. Then on any breath out, as slowly as you would like today, come back to standing tall.

5. Feel the Breath with Fingertip Press

Key Phrases: (1) Longer breaths in *can* be energizing. (2) Long, slow breaths out *can* lower blood pressure.

Opening Cue: Noticing your breath can be a first step in managing how you breathe.

Cues:

1. When you are ready, gently press one shoulder back… Then press the other shoulder back.
2. If you like, put one or both hands over your heart… Put one or both hands over your heart.
3. The suggestion is to practice 5 breaths. Feel the breath in, fingertips press… Feel the breath out, release the press. (*Say 2 times slowly.*) Always breathe in a comfortable way.
   Feel the breath in, fingertips press… Feel the breath out, release. (*Say 3 times slowly.*)
4. If you like, gently move the fingers on one hand or shake that hand… Then gently move the fingers on the other hand or shake that hand.

6. Warrior 1 Flow (Side 1: a/b/c/d; Side 2: a/b/c/e)
A. ACHILLES TENDON AND CALF STRETCH (PHOTOS ON P.246)

Key Phrase: We move slowly so you can "find a better way to move."

Opening Cue: Gentle moving and stretching can lubricate your ankle and knee joints.

Cues:

1. We always do both sides. When you are ready, put one hand on the back of the chair. Step one foot straight back so your heel is off the floor.
2. Gently press one shoulder back… Then press the other shoulder back.
3. Today you may focus on the stretch and keep one hand on the chair. Or today you may want your hand off the chair to focus on building core muscles.

4. The suggestion is to practice this Achilles tendon and calf stretch 3 times. Keeping a slight bend in your front knee protects that knee joint. As YOU breathe in, lift your back heel... As YOU breathe out, gently press the heel toward the floor. (*Say 3 times slowly.*)

B. WARRIOR 1 (PHOTOS ON P.246)

Key Phrase: You can come out of a stretch anytime; you are never stuck.

Opening Cue: Warrior 1 can both stretch and strengthen muscles.

Cues:

1. If you like, bend the front knee a comfortable distance.
2. Stretch one or both arms toward the ceiling, fingers spread wide in warrior 1. You are building core strength as you move to find your balance in this power pose. With your hand on the chair, you can focus on the stretch. (**Variation.**)
3. The suggestion is to hold the stretch for 3 breaths. Hold the stretch... but not the breath. Feel the breath in, fingers stretch... Feel the breath out, fingers release. (*Say 3 times slowly*.)

Variation: For a supported backbend, when you are ready press one or both palms or gentle fists against the sides or back of your hips. Draw your elbows and shoulders back as you arc back a comfortable distance. Today you may want to arc one or both arms overhead.

C. WARRIOR 1 WITH A TWIST

Key Phrase: Different days, different stretches.

Opening Cue: Gentle twists can lengthen the spine and improve circulation.

Cues:

1. When you are ready, make any adjustments in your front knee so you feel strong. Then place your opposite hand on the back of the chair or on your front leg.
2. If you like, move your other hand across to the side or back of your hip. The suggestion is to practice 4 breaths here. Feel the breath in... Feel the breath out. (*Say 4 times slowly.*) When you are ready, come back to standing tall.

D. TIP-TO-TOE STRETCH (*AFTER SIDE 1*)
Cues:

1. When you are ready, stretch one arm to the side or overhead, fingers stretched wide. Then stretch the other arm to the side or overhead, fingers stretched wide.
2. Find your own rhythm as you stretch from tip-to-toe. Take your time with these stretches, stretching one arm and then the other.
3. When you are ready, arms release. (**Repeat a/b/c/e on the other side.**)

E. ANYTIME, ANYWHERE BREATH (*AFTER SIDE 2*)

Key Phrase: Long, slow breaths out *can* lower heart rate, lower blood pressure, and lower muscle tension.

Opening Cue: One way we can manage pain in real-time is by choosing how we breathe.

Cues: You can do the Anytime, Anywhere Breath even when talking with someone.

1. When you are ready, gently press one shoulder back... Then press the other shoulder back. If you like, place one hand on your leg in a way that is comfortable.
2. Let's practice 5 breaths. The suggestion is to take long, slow breaths out. (**Variation 1.**)
   As YOU breathe in, fingers press... As YOU breathe out, release. (*Say 2 times slowly.*)
   Always breathe in a comfortable way.
   On YOUR next breath in, fingers press... As YOU breathe out, release. As YOU breathe in, fingers press... As YOU breathe out, release. (*Say 2 times slowly.*)
3. If you like, gently move the fingers on one hand or shake that hand... Then gently move the fingers on the other hand or shake that hand. (**Variation 2.**)
4. You may want to practice the Anytime, Anywhere Breath later, when you want to change how you are feeling.

Variations: (1) Press your fingers firmly or gently today. **Or** (2) Now if you like, use your other hand and practice saying it 5 times to yourself in your mind, since *you* are always with you. (*Say slowly during this time so there is no "dead air:" Don't rush your words... Don't rush your breath. Take your time with your words... Take your time with your breath.*)

SIXTY- TO NINETY-MINUTE PRACTICES

B. Seated (10 minutes)
1. Get Yourself Set Up
Key Phrases: (1) Anything we do seated, you can do standing or even lying down. (2) You can always find ways to move and to breathe with me.

Opening Cue: Sitting or standing with your shoulders gently pressed back can take pressure off your back.

Cues:

1. Give yourself a few moments to find a comfortable way to sit today, either on a folded blanket or on a chair.
2. Gently press one shoulder back... Then press the other shoulder back.
3. If you like, move from side to side as you settle into your seat. Perhaps move in a circle. Take your time as you move. You may want to circle even more slowly the other way.
4. Make any adjustments to find a more comfortable seat.

2. Physiological Sigh
Key Phrase: Doing the physiological sigh 2 or 3 times can help lower carbon dioxide levels in the blood, which can lower anxiety.

Opening Cue: You can interrupt your stress cycle by choosing how you breathe.

Cues:

1. When you are ready, gently press one shoulder back... Then press the other shoulder back.
2. Let's practice once. Always move and breathe in a comfortable way. When you are ready, practice a deep breath in and stretch your fingers wide. Then breathe in more; perhaps stretch your fingers a little more. Hold that breath as long as you like... Then SIGH it out. The suggestion is to practice 2 more times. (*Say 2 more times.*)
3. If you like, gently move the fingers on one hand or shake that hand... Then gently move the fingers on the other hand or shake that hand.
4. The physiological sigh is a way to practice lowering anxiety in 2 or 3 breaths.

3. Shoulder Rolls (photos on p.254)
Key Phrase: Today you may want to practice long breaths out.

Opening Cue: A long breath out *can* reduce muscle tension.

Cues:

1. The suggestion is to do 3 shoulder rolls forward and 3 shoulder rolls back. As YOU breathe in, shoulders lift... As YOU breathe out, shoulders roll forward and down. (*Say 3 times slowly.*)
Always move in a comfortable way.
2. Now 3 back. As YOU breathe in, shoulders lift... As YOU breathe out, shoulders roll back and down. (*Say 3 times slowly.*)

Variations: (1) After one roll: if you like, move even more slowly on the next two rolls. **Or** (2) After two rolls: if you like, stop halfway down this last roll. Hold the stretch...but not your breath.

4. Core Check (photos on p.248)

Key Phrases: (1) Keeping your shoulders gently pressed back can reduce pain. (2) You can always change the way you are moving; you are never stuck.

Opening Cues: Taking long breaths out when you feel discomfort can interrupt your stress cycle. Building core strength can help keep your spine in alignment. The suggestion is to practice both now as we do Core Check.

Cues:

1. When you are ready, sit forward on your chair or a folded blanket.
2. Gently press one shoulder back... Then press the other shoulder back.
3. Slide your hands back. If you feel any burning, numbness, or tingling, adjust your stretch.
4. Notice your next breath in... On YOUR breath out, release back until you feel some core muscles working. Moving even half an inch or a few centimeters has benefit.
5. Take 2 breaths here if you like. As YOU breathe in, fingers stretch... As YOU breathe out, release. (*Say 2 times slowly.*) When you are ready, come back to sitting tall. That was you building core muscles and "not holding your breath" when feeling some discomfort. You might like to say quietly, "Check."
6. The suggestion is to do this gentle strengthening 4 more times. Notice that one shoulder is still back...and that the other shoulder is back. As YOU breathe in, hands press... As YOU breathe out, release back. Today perhaps lift one leg. (**Adapt variations for your group.**)
7. When you feel muscles working, practice 2 more breaths. As YOU breathe in, fingers stretch... As YOU breathe out, release. (*Say 2 times slowly.*) Come back to sitting tall. "Check." (**Repeat 3 more times.**)

Variations: (1) Lift one or both arms to shoulder height as you release back. **Or** (2) Lift one leg (knee bent or leg straight) as you release back. **Or** (3) Lift both arms and one or both legs as you release back.

5. Feel the Breath with Fingertip Press

Key Phrases: (1) Longer breaths in *can* be energizing. (2) Long, slow breaths out *can* lower blood pressure. (*Or choose one of these phrases based on what fits the needs of the class.*)

Opening Cue: Noticing your breath can be a first step in managing how you breathe.

Cues:

1. When you are ready, gently press one shoulder back... Then press the other shoulder back.
   If you like, put one or both hands over your heart... Put one or both hands over your heart.
2. The suggestion is to practice 5 breaths. Feel the breath in, fingertips press... Feel the breath out, release the press. (*Say 2 times slowly.*)
   Always breathe in a comfortable way.
   Feel the breath in, fingertips press... Feel the breath out, release. (*Say 3 times slowly.*)
3. If you like, gently move the fingers on one hand or shake that hand... Then gently move the fingers on the other hand or shake that hand.

C. Lying Down (15 minutes)
1. Get Yourself Set Up

Key Phrases: (1) Anything we do lying down, you can do seated or standing. (2) You can always find ways to move and to breathe with me.

Opening Cue: Major muscles that usually work to hold us up can release when we lie down.

Cues: Give yourself a few moments to get yourself set up. You can make adjustments; you are never stuck.

1. You may want a rolled-up blanket, towel, or mat under your knees before you lie back.
2. Today, you also may want a small roll (washcloth or towel) under your neck for support.

2. The Noticing Breath

Key Phrase: Long, slow breaths out *can* lower heart rate, lower blood pressure, and lower muscle tension.

Opening Cue: One way we can manage pain in real-time is by choosing how we breathe.

Cues: Notice if you have any area in which you feel discomfort—either physical or emotional. Or pick an area on which to practice—your knee, perhaps.

1. The Noticing Breath is 5 breaths. The suggestion is long, slow breaths out if that is comfortable for you today.
2. When you are ready, gently press one shoulder back... Then press the other shoulder back.
3. On YOUR breath in, notice that area of discomfort... On YOUR breath out, keep noticing. (*Say 2 times slowly.*) Instead of ignoring the discomfort, the suggestion is to keep noticing it as you breathe.
   On YOUR NEXT breath in, notice that area... On YOUR breath out, keep noticing.
   On YOUR breath in, notice that area... On YOUR breath out, keep noticing. (*Say 2 times slowly.*)
4. If you like, gently move the fingers on one hand or shake that hand. Then gently move the fingers on the other hand or shake that hand.
5. You may want to practice the Noticing Breath later, when you want to interrupt your stress cycle.

3. Gentle Twist with Knees (photos on p.258)

Key Phrases: (1) We move slowly so you have time "to find a better way to move." (2) There is no place you are trying to go with the stretch.

Opening Cue: A gentle twist can create space between the spinal bones by gently stretching the outer hip muscles that can pull on the spine.

Cues:

1. When you are ready, put your feet on the floor under your knees. Extend your arms, palms up or down, in a comfortable way.
2. Slowly move your knees from side to side, noticing what feels like a comfortable stretch today.
3. You can add to the stretch by crossing one knee over the other. We always do both sides. (**Variation.**) If you like, continue to move slowly from side to side.

4. The suggestion is to find one gentle twist to hold. Hold the stretch... but not the breath. Let's practice 2 breaths. Feel the breath in... Feel the breath out. (*Say 2 times slowly.*)
5. If you like, cross your knees the other way and find your own rhythm as you move.
6. Again, the suggestion is to find one gentle twist to hold. Hold the stretch...but not the breath. Let's take 2 breaths. Feel the breath in... Feel the breath out. (*Say 2 times slowly.*)
7. When you are ready, uncross your legs, pull them in, and rock from side to side. (**Repeat on the other side.**)

Variation: If you like, slowly move your knees to one side and look the opposite way for a full spinal twist.

4. Bridge Flow (a/b/c) (photos on p.259)
A. RAISING YOUR HEART
Key Phrase: Use the pieces of the stretch that feel comfortable for you today.

Opening Cue: Gently lifting and tucking your tailbone as you are lying down can release some muscle tension and increase circulation.

Cues: The suggestion is to practice Raising Your Heart 3 times.

1. When you are ready, put your feet on the floor, under your knees.
2. As YOU breathe in, press down on your hips and shoulders, gently raising your heart as you arch your back a comfortable distance.
3. If you like, press your shoulders in toward your spine. Keep breathing in a comfortable way.
4. Notice your next breath in... On YOUR *next* breath out, slowly release, pull your legs in, and wrap your arms around your shins (or backs of your legs). Press as firmly as is comfortable for you today. If you like, we can practice another 2 Raising Your Heart flows. (**Repeat 2 more times.**)

B. BRIDGE LIFT AND RELEASE
Key Phrase: Long, slow breaths out can lower heart rate, lower blood pressure, and lower muscle tension.

Opening Cue: Moving in this bridge flow can strengthen core muscles.

Cues: When you are ready, put your feet on the floor under your knees again. The suggestion is to practice bridge lift and release 3 times.

1. As YOU breathe in, press down on your feet and gently lift your hips, any distance. (**Variation.**)

2. On YOUR next breath out, slowly release down and pull your knees in. Perhaps wrap your arms around your shins or backs of your legs and press as firmly as is comfortable. (**Repeat 3 times.**)
3. Still in a wrap, if you like, practice 3 breaths. You may want to practice long, slow breaths out. As you breathe in, fingers press... As you breathe out, fingers release. (*Say 2 times slowly.*)

Variation: With your hips still lifted, extend your arms overhead, hands on the floor behind you. If you like, take 2 breaths here. Feel the breath in... Feel the breath out. (*Say 2 times slowly.*)

C. SIDE-TO-SIDE ROCKING

Key Phrase: Different days, different stretches.

Opening Cue: Gently moving as you are lying down can massage connective tissue and reduce muscle tension.

Cues:

1. When you are ready, pull both knees in...perhaps wrap your hands around the fronts of the shins or backs of the legs.
2. The suggestion is to gently rock from side to side. You may want to wiggle your toes as you rock. Move your feet in any way that feels comfortable for you today.
3. Take your time with these gentle stretches. (**Variation.**)
4. Notice your next breath in... As YOU breathe out, release one leg to the floor. Notice your next breath in... As you breathe out, release the other leg to the floor.

Variation: Cross ankles as you rock. Then reverse and continue rocking.

D. Final Stretch (15 minutes) (see p.218)
1. Get Yourself Set Up

2. Final Stretch: A Body-Based, Guided Meditation

E. Make a Plan

F. Extras
1. Time Adjustments
Running Out of Time? After lying down gentle twist with knees, do one bridge flow and go to Final Stretch.

2. Theme Variation: Little Changes
After you have done this practice several times, you can offer this idea at the beginning and mention it a few times during the practice:

> Today, you might want to do the stretches in a different way. You can make little changes as we move and breathe.

3. Ideas to extend to a 90-minute practice
A. SEATED: * SHOULDER SUITE (P.126); * TIP-TO-TOE STRETCH (P.244)

B. LYING DOWN: * TIP-TO-TOE STRETCH (P.258); * SHOULDER STRETCH (PP.180–1); * #4 STRETCH (P.251); * THE NOTICING BREATH (P.110); * EXTENDED MAKE A PLAN (P.220)

II. STRETCH, BREATHE, REST, AND RESTORE (STANDING/SEATED/LYING DOWN)
Note: Please review In Case You Missed It... (p.101)

A. Standing (5 minutes)
1. Tip-to-Toe Stretch (photos on p.243)
Key Phrase: When we do not move, tight muscles can press on nerves and joints.

Opening Cue: As Moshé Feldenkrais said, "There isn't a right way to move; there is a better way to move."

Cues:

1. When you are ready, stretch one arm to the side or overhead, fingers stretched wide in the Tip-to-Toe Stretch.
2. Then stretch the other arm, either to the side or overhead, fingers stretched wide.
3. Find your own rhythm as you stretch one arm and then the other. We move slowly so you can "find a better way to move" toward a healthier spine. (**Variations.**)
4. When you are ready, put your hands on your hips.
   If you like, lift one heel and press on the toes. Then lift the other heel and press on the toes. Let's practice that toe stretch two more times. (*Say 2 times slowly.*)

Variations: (1) Today you may like to arc one arm overhead and then the other. Find your own rhythm as you move. **Or** (2) As you stretch one arm, lift the heel on the other side. Find your own rhythm as you stretch the arm and lift the other heel. When you are ready, stretch one arm and lift the heel on the same side. Move in a comfortable way, stretching and lifting. Then if you like, practice the way that was more of a challenge.

2. Wide-Legged Add-On (photos on p.245)

Key Phrase: Moving even half an inch or a few centimeters has benefits; it means muscles are not getting tighter.

Opening Cue: Another way we can manage pain is with gentle stretches to reduce pressure on nerves and lubricate joints.

Cues:

1. When you are ready, step your feet apart, hands on your hips as we do the wide-legged add-on. (**Variation.**)
2. In whatever way feels comfortable, move one hip to one side... Then move the other hip to the other side. We move slowly so you can "find a better way to move."
3. Today you may like to add lifting your shoulder in a gentle arc as you move to one side... Then lift the other shoulder in a gentle arc as you move the other hip to the side. Find your own rhythm as you move from side to side. Take your time as you move.
4. When you are ready, come back to standing tall. If you like, gently *stretch* the fingers on one hand or shake that hand... Then gently *stretch* the fingers or shake the other hand.

Variation: Today you may want to roll from the inside edges to the outside edges of your feet... Roll from the inside to the outside edges in any way that is comfortable for you today.

3. Feel the Breath

Key Phrases: (1) Longer breaths in *can* be energizing. (2) Long, slow breaths out *can* lower blood pressure. (*Or choose one of these phrases based on what fits the needs of the class.*)

Opening Cue: You can interrupt your stress cycle by choosing how you breathe.

Cues:

1. When you are ready, gently press one shoulder back... Then press the other shoulder back.

SIXTY- TO NINETY-MINUTE PRACTICES

2. If you like, put one or both hands over your heart... Put one or both hands over your heart.
3. The suggestion is to practice 5 breaths. Today you may like to practice long breaths out.
   Feel the breath in... Feel the breath out. (*Say 2 times slowly.*)
   Always breathe in a comfortable way.
   Feel the breath in... Feel the breath out. (*Say 3 times slowly.*)
4. If you like, gently move the fingers on one hand or shake that hand... Then gently move the fingers on the other hand or shake that hand.

B. Seated (15 minutes)
1. Get Yourself Set Up
Key Phrase: Anything we do seated, you can do standing or even lying down.

Opening Cue: Sitting or standing with your shoulders gently pressed back can take pressure off your back.

Cues:

1. Give yourself a few moments to find a comfortable way to sit today, either on a folded blanket or on a chair.
2. Gently press one shoulder back, and then press the other shoulder back.
3. If you like, move from side to side as you settle into your seat. Perhaps move in a circle. Take your time as you move. You may want to circle the other way even more slowly.
4. Make any adjustments to find a more comfortable seat.

2. The Wave Breath (photos on p.262)
Key Phrases: (1) Long, slow breaths out *can* lower blood pressure. (2) Longer breaths in *can* be energizing.

Opening Cue: You can interrupt your stress cycle by choosing how you breathe.

Cues:

1. Notice if your shoulders are still gently pressed back.
2. The suggestion is to take 5 breaths as we practice the Wave Breath.
   As YOU breathe in, hands lift (*palms up*). As YOU breathe out, release (*palms down*). (*Say 2 times slowly.*)
   Always breathe in a comfortable way. On YOUR next breath in, hands lift... As YOU breathe out, release.

As YOU breathe in, hands lift... As YOU breathe out, release. (*Say 2 times slowly.*)
3. If you like, gently move the fingers on one hand or shake that hand... Then gently move the fingers on the other hand or shake that hand.

3. Neck and Shoulder Suite (a/b/c) (photos on p.255)

A. NECK MASSAGE

Key Phrase: Even small stretches have benefits.

Opening Cue: Gently massaging muscles as you sit can reduce physical and emotional tension.

Cues:

1. The suggestion is to use one hand to massage the back of your neck, or if it's more comfortable for you today, the fronts of your shoulders. (**Variation.**)
2. Today you may want to: (*Slowly cue and do each one.*)
   a. Use one or both hands.
   b. Gently tuck your chin and move from side to side as you massage.
   c. Massage the base of your neck/top of your back.
   d. Gently lift and lower your chin as you massage.

Variation: Use a gentle or firm massage in a way that feels comfortable for you today.

B. CHIN LIFTS AND PENDULUM

Key Phrases: (1) You may be moving an inch or a few centimeters, and that has benefits. (2) Some days, visualizing the stretch may be more helpful.

Opening Cue: The head weighs about 10 pounds or 4.5 kilograms. Gently stretching neck muscles can relieve some tension and pain.

Cues:

1. The suggestion is to practice this *slow* stretch 3 times. As YOU breathe in, chin slowly lifts... As YOU breathe out, chin slowly releases. (*Say 3 times slowly.*)
2. With your chin still released, move your chin from side to side, like a pendulum. Take your time with each slow stretch.

C. NECK AND SHOULDER STRETCHES

Key Phrase: You can change how you are stretching any time; you are never stuck.

Opening Cue: Gently stretching muscles around the neck and shoulders as you sit can reduce some neck and back pain.

Cues:

1. We always do both sides. The suggestion is to gently release your *left* ear toward your *left* shoulder. Moving even half an inch or a few centimeters has benefit.
2. When you are ready, move your *right* shoulder, practicing each of these slow stretches 3 times:
   a. Press your shoulder forward... Then press it back. (*Say 3 times slowly.*)
   b. As YOU breathe in, lift that shoulder... As YOU breathe out, press that shoulder down as firmly as is comfortable for you today. If you like, hold this press for 2 more breaths. Hold the press...but not your breath. Feel the breath in... Feel the breath out. (*Say 2 times slowly.*) **(Repeat 2 more times.)**
   c. Now roll this shoulder forward 3 times in a comfortable way. Take your time with this slow stretch. When you are ready, roll this shoulder back 3 times. Again, take your time as you "find a better way to move."
3. When you are ready, come back to sitting tall. If you like, let's practice 2 more chin lifts. On YOUR breath in, chin slowly lifts... On YOUR breath out, chin slowly releases. (*Say 2 times slowly.*) **(Repeat #1-3 on the other side.)**

4. Shoulder Rolls (photos on p.254)

Key Phrase: Today you may want to practice long breaths out.

Opening Cue: A long breath out can reduce muscle tension.

Cues:

1. The suggestion is to do 3 shoulder rolls forward and 3 shoulder rolls back. As YOU breathe in, shoulders lift... As YOU breathe out, shoulders roll forward and down. (*Say 3 times slowly.*) Always move in a comfortable way.
2. Now 3 back. As YOU breathe in, shoulders lift... As YOU breathe out, shoulders roll back and down. (*Say 3 times slowly.*)

Variations: (1) After one roll: if you like, move even more slowly on the next two rolls. **Or** (2) After two rolls: if you like, stop halfway down the next roll. Hold the stretch...but not your breath.

5. Finger Stretch Breath

Key Phrases: (1) Longer breaths in *can* be energizing. (2) Long, slow breaths out *can* lower heart rate, lower blood pressure, and lower muscle tension.

Opening Cue: One way we can manage pain in real-time is by choosing how we breathe.

Cues: In Finger Stretch Breath, the suggestion is to stretch your fingers about half an inch or a few centimeters. (**Variations.**)

1. When you are ready, gently press one shoulder back... Then press the other shoulder back. If you like, let's practice 5 breaths.
2. As YOU breathe in, fingers stretch... As YOU breathe out, release. (*Say 2 times slowly.*)
   Always breathe in a comfortable way. On YOUR next breath in, fingers stretch... As YOU breathe out, release.
   As YOU breathe in, fingers stretch... As YOU breathe out, release. (*Say 2 times slowly.*)
3. If you like, gently move the fingers on one hand or shake that hand...then gently move the fingers on the other hand or shake that hand.

Variations: (1) Stretch your fingers just enough to notice the stretch. **Or** (2) Stretch your fingers as wide as you would like today. **Or** (3) Perhaps stretch your fingers in a different way today.

6. Classic Twist with Cat/Cow (photos on p.242)

Key Phrase: There is no place you are trying to go with a stretch.

Opening Cue: The suggestion is to practice one more seated twist to create space between spinal bones with gentle stretches.

Cues:

1. Gently press one shoulder back... Then press the other shoulder back. If you like, tap your *fingertips* on your legs.
2. We always do both sides. On YOUR next breath in, press down on hands and feet. As YOU breathe out, bring your hands around to one side. (**Variation.**)
3. The suggestion is to take 4 breaths here. As YOU breathe in, hands press.

As YOU breathe out, release the press. (*Say 4 times slowly.*) When you are ready, come back to facing front. If you like, tap your *fingertips* on your legs.
4. Before we do the other side, the suggestion is to practice seated cat/cow 2 times.
5. As YOU breathe in, chin lifts...shoulders back...rock forward.
As YOU breathe out, chin tucks...shoulders forward...rock back a comfortable distance. Always move and breathe in a comfortable way. On YOUR next breath in, chin lifts...shoulders back...rock forward. As YOU breathe out, chin tucks...shoulders forward...rock back a comfortable distance.
6. When you are ready, come back to sitting tall. (**Repeat on the other side.**)

Variation: When it feels easy to breathe in the twist, you may want to look forward for a full spinal twist. If you like, practice 4 breaths here.

C. Lying Down (25 minutes)
1. Get Yourself Set Up
Key Phrases: (1) Anything we do lying down, you can do seated or standing. (2) You can always find ways to move and to breathe with me.

Opening Cue: Major muscles that usually work to hold us up can release when we lie down.

Cues: Give yourself a few moments to get set up. You can make adjustments; you are never stuck.

1. You may want a rolled-up blanket, towel, or mat under your knees before you lie back.
2. Today, you also may want a small roll (washcloth or towel) under your neck for support.

2. The Noticing Breath
Key Phrase: Long, slow breaths out *can* lower heart rate, lower blood pressure, and lower muscle tension.

Opening Cue: You can interrupt your stress cycle by choosing how you breathe.

Cues: Notice if you have any area in which you feel discomfort—either physical or emotional. Or today pick an area on which to practice—your knee, perhaps.

1. The Noticing Breath is 5 breaths. The suggestion is long, slow breaths out if that is comfortable for you today.
2. When you are ready, gently press one shoulder back... Then press the other shoulder back.
3. On YOUR breath in, notice that area of discomfort... On YOUR breath out, keep noticing. (*Say 2 times slowly.*) Instead of ignoring the discomfort, the suggestion is to keep noticing it as you breathe.

    On YOUR next breath in, notice that area... On YOUR breath out, keep noticing.

    On YOUR breath in, notice that area... On YOUR breath out, keep noticing. (*Say 2 times slowly.*)
4. If you like, gently move the fingers on one hand or shake that hand. Then gently move the fingers on the other hand or shake that hand.
5. You may want to practice the Noticing Breath later, when you want to interrupt your stress cycle.

3. Bridge Flow (a/b/c) (photos on p.259)

A. RAISING YOUR HEART

Key Phrase: Use the pieces of the stretch that feel comfortable for you today.

Opening Cue: When you are lying down, stretching can release some muscle tension and increase circulation.

Cues: The suggestion is to practice Raising Your Heart 3 times.

1. When you are ready, put your feet on the floor under your knees.
2. As YOU breathe in, press down on your hips and shoulders, gently raising your heart as you arch your back a comfortable distance.
3. If you like, press your shoulders in toward your spine. Keep breathing in a comfortable way.
4. Notice your next breath in... On YOUR *next* breath out, slowly release, pull your legs in, and wrap your arms around your shins (or backs of your legs). Press as firmly as is comfortable for you today. If you like, we can practice another 2 Raising Your Heart flows. (**Repeat 2 more times.**)

B. BRIDGE LIFT AND RELEASE

Key Phrase: Long, slow breaths out *can* lower heart rate, lower blood pressure, and lower muscle tension.

Opening Cue: Moving in this bridge flow can strengthen core muscles.

SIXTY- TO NINETY-MINUTE PRACTICES

Cues: When you are ready, put your feet on the floor under your knees again. The suggestion is to practice bridge lift and release 3 times.

1. As YOU breathe in, press down on your feet and gently lift your hips, any distance. (**Variation.**)
2. On YOUR next breath out, slowly release down and pull your knees in. Perhaps wrap your arms around your shins or backs of your legs and press as firmly as is comfortable. (**Repeat 3 times.**)
3. Still in a wrap, if you like, take 3 breaths. You may want to practice long, slow breaths out. As you breathe in, fingers press... As you breathe out, fingers release. (*Say 2 times slowly.*)

Variation: With your hips still lifted, extend your arms overhead, hands on the floor behind you. If you like, take 2 breaths here. Feel the breath in... Feel the breath out. (*Say 2 times slowly.*)

C. SIDE-TO-SIDE ROCKING
Key Phrase: Different days, different stretches.

Opening Cue: Gently moving can massage connective tissue and reduce muscle tension.

Cues:

1. With your knees still pulled in, perhaps gently rock from side to side. If you like, wiggle your toes as you rock. Take your time with the stretches.
2. Give yourself a moment to move your feet in any way that feels comfortable for you today. (**Variation.**)
3. When you are ready, notice your next breath in... On YOUR breath out, slowly release the one leg to the floor.
4. Notice your next breath in... On YOUR breath out, slowly release the other leg to the floor.

Variation: Cross your ankles as you rock. If you like, cross the other way and continue rocking.

4. Gentle Twist with Knees (photos on p.258)
Key Phrases: (1) We move slowly so you have time "to find a better way to move." (2) There is no place you are trying to go with the stretch.

Opening Cue: A gentle twist can create space between the spinal bones by gently stretching the outer hip muscles that can pull on the spine.

Cues:

1. When you are ready, put your feet on the floor under your knees. Extend your arms, palms up or down, in a comfortable way.
2. Slowly move your knees from side to side, noticing what feels like a comfortable stretch today.
3. You can add to the stretch by crossing one knee over the other. We always do both sides. (**Variation.**) If you like, continue to move slowly from side to side.
4. The suggestion is to find one gentle twist to hold. Hold the stretch… but not the breath. Let's practice 2 breaths. Feel the breath in… Feel the breath out. (*Say 2 times slowly.*)
5. If you like, cross your knees the other way and find your own rhythm as you move.
6. Again, the suggestion is to find one gentle twist to hold. Hold the stretch…but not the breath. Let's take 2 breaths. Feel the breath in… Feel the breath out. (*Say 2 times slowly.*)
7. When you are ready, uncross your legs, pull them in, and rock from side to side. (**Repeat on the other side.**)

Variation: If you like, slowly move your knees to one side and look the opposite way for a full spinal twist.

5. Feel the Breath with Fingertip Press

Key Phrase: Longer breaths in *can* be energizing.

Opening Cue: Noticing your breath can be a first step in managing how you breathe.

Cues:

1. When you are ready, gently press one shoulder back… Then press the other shoulder back.
2. If you like, put one or both hands over your heart… Put one or both hands over your heart.
3. The suggestion is to practice 5 breaths. (**Variation 1.**) Feel the breath in, fingertips press… Feel the breath out, release the press. (*Say 2 times slowly.*)
   Always breathe in a comfortable way.
   Feel the breath in, fingertips press… Feel the breath out, release. (*Say 3 times slowly.*)
4. If you like, gently move the fingers on one hand or shake that hand… Then gently move the fingers on the other hand or shake that hand.

Variations: (1) If you like, after you feel the breath in, pause long enough to notice the pause, then... Feel the breath out... **Or** (2) If you like, after you feel the breath out, pause long enough to notice the pause, then feel the breath in...

6. Hip-to-Toe Stretches (a/b/c/d/e/f) (photos on p.261)

A. TOES, FOOT, AND ANKLE 1

Key Phrase: Small movements have benefits—even half an inch or a few centimeters.

Opening Cue: Gentle stretches can take pressure off joints and improve circulation.

Cues:

1. We always do both sides. When you are ready, rest one leg on the floor and bend your other knee.
2. Wrap your hands around the front of your shin or the back of your leg.
3. The suggestion is to slowly move that foot in a circle. When you are ready, circle the other way.
4. If you like, stretch all your toes on both feet 3 times. On YOUR breath in, stretch your toes... As YOU breathe out, release. (*Say 3 times slowly.*)

B. TOES, FOOT, AND ANKLE 2

Key Phrase: Put as much muscle energy into the stretch as feels comfortable for you today.

Opening Cue: We move slowly to practice "finding a better way to move."

Cues:

1. When you are ready, begin to move that foot as if pressing a gas pedal. Slowly press the toes away and then pull the toes toward your shin. Now if you like, hold each stretch for 2 breaths. Hold the stretch...but not the breath. Press your toes away. Feel the breath in... Feel the breath out. (*Say 2 times slowly.*) Then pull the toes toward you. Feel the breath in... Feel the breath out. (*Say 2 times slowly.*)
2. If you like, stretch all your toes 3 times again. As YOU breathe in, stretch your toes... As YOU breathe out, release. (*Say 3 times slowly.*)

C. KNEE STRETCH (PHOTO ON P.261)

Key Phrase: Always move in a way that is comfortable for you today.

Opening Cue: Small, gentle stretches can keep the knee joints healthy and lubricated, which can reduce pain.

Cues:

1. Hold the top part of your leg (femur) steady as you circle the foot, as if drawing on the wall in front of you. (**Variation.**) The gentle movement can massage tendons and ligaments, as well as lengthen muscles. It can be any size circle or any shape that is comfortable.
2. When you are ready, slowly move in the other direction.

Variation: If you feel like being silly today, imagine drawing with a color crayon that makes you feel silly.

D. SPIRAL HIP STRETCH

Key Phrase: Different days, different stretches.

Opening Cue: Moving slowly allows you to gently stretch and lubricate the hip joints.

Cues:

1. When you are ready, release your hands to your sides, knee still bent as we do the spiral hip stretch. Begin to move that knee in a circle or shape that feels comfortable. (**Variation.**)
2. Perhaps today sweep that leg across to the other side and then pull it toward you making a different spiral. Take your time with these stretches to lubricate the hip joint. When you are ready, circle the other way.

Variation: If you feel like being silly today, imagine you are drawing on the ceiling with a color crayon that makes you feel silly.

E. OUTER HIP STRETCH/TWIST

Key Phrase: There is no place you are trying to go with a stretch.

Opening Cue: Let's gently stretch the outer hip muscles and the spine.

Cues:

1. When you are ready, place your foot above or next to the knee on the other leg. Gently draw that knee across. Even small movements have benefits.
2. If you like, look the opposite way for a full spinal twist. Stay here for 4 more breaths if that is comfortable for you today. Feel the breath in… Feel the breath out. (*Say 4 times slowly.*)

Variation: For these 4 breaths: As YOU breathe in, fingers press. As YOU breathe out, release the press.

F. BACK RELEASE 1

Key Phrase: Use the pieces of the stretch that feel comfortable for you today.

Opening Cue: The suggestion is to take long, slow breaths out if that is comfortable for you today.

Cues: When you are ready, put both feet on the floor under your knees. Let's practice this back release 3 times.

1. As YOU breathe in, press down on your feet and gently lift your hips, any distance...
   As YOU breathe out, slowly release down, and on the *same* long, slow breath out, pull your knees in and wrap your arms around your shins or backs of your legs. (*Say 3 times slowly.*)
2. Now, with your arms still around your legs, let's practice 3 breaths. As YOU breathe in, fingers press... As YOU breathe out, fingers release. (*Say 3 times slowly.*)
3. Notice your next breath in... As YOU breathe out, slowly release one leg to the floor. Notice your next breath in... As YOU breathe out, slowly release the other leg to the floor. (**Repeat a/b/c/d/e/f on the other side.**)

D. Final Stretch (15 minutes) (see p.218)
1. Get Yourself Set Up (photo on p.258)

2. Final Stretch: A Body-Based, Guided Meditation

E. Make a Plan

F. Extras
1. Time Adjustments
Running Out of Time? After lying down and Feel the Breath, go to Final Stretch.

2. Theme Variation: The Pause
After you have done this practice several times, you can offer this idea at the beginning and mention it a few times during the practice:

Today, you might want to notice if you pause between the breath in and the breath out. You don't need to change it, unless you want to play with pausing and noticing it.

3. Ideas to extend to a 90-minute practice
A. SEATED: * SHOULDER SUITE (P.126); * TIP-TO-TOE STRETCH (P.244)

B. LYING DOWN: * TIP-TO-TOE STRETCH (P.258); * SHOULDER STRETCH (PP.180–1); * #4 STRETCH (P.251); * THE NOTICING BREATH (P.110)

C. FINAL STRETCH: * EXTENDED MAKE A PLAN (P.220)

C. "Final Stretch:" A Body-Based, Guided Meditation (15 minutes)
1. GET YOURSELF SET UP

(*This setup is the one place I demonstrate all the options.*) Give yourself a few moments to get yourself set up. Anything we do lying down, you can do seated if that is more comfortable for you today. You can make adjustments; you are never stuck.

1. If you are sitting in a chair, you may want a rolled-up mat or blanket behind your low back. If you are sitting on the floor, perhaps sit on a blanket.
2. Before you lie back, you may want a rolled-up blanket, towel, or mat under your knees. You also may want to put another rolled-up blanket or mat lengthwise behind you so when you lie back your head and back are supported.
3. A small roll (washcloth or towel) under your neck can give more support.

2. FINAL STRETCH: A BODY-BASED, GUIDED MEDITATION (10 MINUTES)

In Final Stretch we practice tightening muscles and then releasing them. Only tighten your muscles in a comfortable way. If you like, on YOUR next breath in, close your hand. As YOU breathe out, release. The suggestion is to take long, slow breaths out that *can* lower heart rate, lower blood pressure, and lower muscle tension. Now if you like, on YOUR next breath in, close your other hand. Even a subtle movement has benefits. On YOUR breath out, release. Eyes open or eyes closed, your choice. I keep my eyes open so I can let you know if someone joins us. We always do both sides. I start on the left as a point of reference.

1. When YOU breathe in, close your left hand... As YOU breathe out, release.

SIXTY- TO NINETY-MINUTE PRACTICES

As YOU breathe in, close your hand and tighten your forearm... As YOU breathe out, release.

Always move and breathe in a comfortable way.

As YOUR next breath in, tighten your shoulder... As YOU breathe out, release.

As YOU breathe in, tighten the muscles around your left hip... As YOU breathe out, release.

Now we can tighten the left side of the back, or visualize that you are... Let's practice 3 times.

On YOUR next breath in, tighten the left side of your back... As YOU breathe out, release. (*Say 3 times slowly.*)

On YOUR next breath in, press down on your left heel... As YOU breathe out, release.

2. Now keep breathing as you tighten every muscle you would like on your left side... Perhaps your jaw...shoulder...forearm...hand...left side of your back...hip...and leg.

    When the muscles are as tight as you would like them to be *today*, use YOUR next breath out to release... Perhaps your jaw...shoulder...forearm...hand...left side of your back...hip...and leg.

    Notice YOUR next breath in, chest and belly lift...

    As YOU breathe out, feel your left side fully supported.

    Notice YOUR next breath in, chest and belly lift...

    As YOU breathe out, feel your left side get heavy.

3. Before we do the other side, make any adjustments so you are comfortable for the next few minutes...you are never stuck. (**Repeat slowly on the other side.**)

4. If you like, put one or both hands over your heart...put one or both hands over your heart. Let's practice 5 breaths. Feel the breath in... Feel the breath out. Feel the breath in... Feel the breath out. Now if you like, say the next 3 to yourself in your mind, because *you* are always with you. (*Say slowly during this time to avoid "dead air:" Don't rush your words... Don't rush your breath. Take your time with your words... Take your time with your breath.*)

5. As you are ready, begin to put more effort into your breath in, if that is comfortable for you today. A longer breath in *can* be energizing.

    If you like, extend your arms overhead, hands on the floor behind you. Take up space as you stretch your fingers wide, stretch your toes, and keep taking longer breaths in if that is comfortable for you today.

    As you are ready, gently bend your knees and roll onto your right side, in the interest of personal space, so you are facing away from each other.

6. With your eyes still closed if you like, come up to a comfortable seat. Gently press one shoulder back, and then press the other shoulder back. Let's practice three breaths. As you breathe in, fingers stretch…as you breathe out, release. (*Say 3 times slowly.*)
Give yourself a moment to notice if you met your intention for today… whatever reason you came to practice today. Were you able to make that happen for yourself?

3. MAKE A PLAN

1. Let's end by making a plan to use later in the day or in the night when you want to change how you are feeling. Next time you start to feel pain or discomfort, you can have a 1- to 2-minute plan ready to go.
2. If you like, choose one breath we did today. We did: (*list the breathwork from today's practice*). A long breath out *can* lower blood pressure. So, now you have a 1-minute breath to do.
3. If you like, add one stretch you might like to do again—maybe shoulder rolls or a neck stretch. You now have a 2-minute plan to manage your pain.
4. You also may like to say Final Stretch to yourself to get to sleep or to get back to sleep.

(See www.greentreeyoga.org/pain-management-resources for handouts, the MP3, and other support materials.)

To extend Make a Plan, give time to take 2 breaths to practice the breath they chose. Then they can do (or visualize doing) the stretch they chose. The plan is ready to go.

III. GENTLY MOVING TOWARD A HEALTHIER SPINE (STANDING/SEATED/LYING DOWN)

Note: Before you teach, please review In Case You Missed It… (p.101)

A. Standing (15 minutes)
1. Tip-to-Toe Stretch (photos on p.243)
Key Phrase: Lengthening the spine with the Tip-to-Toe Stretch is one way for you to move toward a healthier spine.

Opening Cue: As Moshé Feldenkrais said, "There isn't a right way to move; there is a better way to move."

SIXTY- TO NINETY-MINUTE PRACTICES

Cues:

1. The suggestion is to stretch one arm to the side or overhead, fingers stretched wide in the Tip-to-Toe Stretch.
2. Then stretch the other arm, either to the side or overhead, fingers stretched wide.
3. Find your own rhythm as you stretch one arm and then the other. We move slowly so you can "find a better way to move" toward a healthier spine. (**Variation.**)
4. When you are ready, put your hands on your hips.
   If you like, lift one heel and press on the toes. Then lift the other heel and press on the toes. Let's create space between the toe joints two more times. (*Say 2 times slowly.*)

Variation: Today you may like to grasp one wrist to help stretch the other arm toward the ceiling. Then grasp the other wrist and stretch toward the ceiling.

2. Feel the Breath

Key Phrases: (1) A long, slow breath out *can* lower heart rate, lower blood pressure, and lower muscle tension. (2) A longer breath in *can* be energizing.

Opening Cue: Noticing your breath can be a first step in managing how you breathe.

Cues:

1. When you are ready, gently press one shoulder back... Then press the other shoulder back.
2. If you like, put one or both hands over your heart... Put one or both hands over your heart.
3. The suggestion is to practice 5 breaths.
   Feel the breath in... Feel the breath out. (*Say 2 times slowly.*)
   Always breathe in a comfortable way.
   Feel the breath in... Feel the breath out. (*Say 3 times slowly.*)
4. If you like, gently stretch the fingers on one hand or shake that hand... Then gently stretch the fingers on the other hand or shake that hand.

3. Side-to-Side (Lateral) Stretches (a/b)

A. CRESCENT STRETCH (PHOTO ON P.245)

Key Phrase: You can make any stretch as gentle or intense or you need today.

Opening Cue: Side-to-side (lateral) stretches are two more ways for you to move toward a healthier spine when you are standing.

Cues:

1. We always do both sides. When you are ready, put your hands on your hips. Then, lift or gently arc one shoulder. Today you may want to arc that arm overhead. If you like, stretch your fingers wide. When you are ready, gently lift and arc on the other side. That's 1 set. Find your own rhythm lifting and gently arcing one shoulder or one arm and then the other as you do 2 more sets. Notice if one side feels different than the other. (**Variation.**)
2. The suggestion is to finish by holding each stretch for 2 breaths. As you lift and gently arc to one side, hold the stretch…but not your breath. Feel the breath in… Feel the breath out. (*Say 2 times slowly.*) When you are ready, lift and gently arc to the other side. Hold the stretch…but not your breath. Feel the breath in… Feel the breath out. (*Say 2 times slowly.*)
3. Now if you like, gently move the fingers on one hand or shake that hand… Then gently move the fingers on the other hand or shake that hand.

Variation: Today you may like to grasp your wrist as you arc one arm overhead. Find your own rhythm as you move from side to side.

B. WIDE-LEGGED ADD-ON (PHOTOS ON P.245)

Key Phrase: Moving even half an inch or a few centimeters has benefits; it means muscles are not getting tighter.

Opening Cue: Gentle side-to-side stretches as you move toward a healthier spine can reduce pressure on nerves and lubricate joints.

Cues:

1. When you are ready, step your feet apart, hands on your hips as we do the wide-legged add-on. (**Variation.**)
2. In whatever way feels comfortable, move one hip to one side… Then move the other hip to the other side. We move slowly so you can "find a better way to move."
3. Today you may like to add lifting your shoulder in a gentle arc as you move to one side… Then lift the other shoulder in a gentle arc as you move the other hip to the side. Find your own rhythm as you move from side to side. Take your time as you move.

4. When you are ready, come back to standing tall. If you like, gently *stretch* the fingers on one hand or shake that hand... Then gently *stretch* the fingers or shake the other hand.

Variation: Today you may want to roll from the inside edges to the outside edges of your feet... Roll from the inside to the outside edges in any way that is comfortable for you today.

4. Kitchen Stretch (a/b/c/b) (photos on pp.249–250)

A. SETUP

Key Phrase: Long, slow breaths out can reduce muscle tension.

Opening Cue: Gently stretching muscles can move you toward a healthier spine.

Cues:

1. Let's practice 3 moves to protect your back and knees as you bend forward. Gently press your shoulders back, press hips back a small amount, and keep a slight bend in your knees.
2. The suggestion is to interlace your fingers and rest your forearms on the back of the chair. If you draw your elbows in so they line up your shoulders, you won't be hanging on your shoulder joints. (**Variation.**)
3. When you are ready, release forward a comfortable distance as we practice Kitchen Stretch.

Variation: Today perhaps try a different setup—pressing your palms together or bending your elbows and lifting your hands toward the ceiling.

B. STRONG AND STEADY

Key Phrase: Long, slow breaths out can reduce muscle tension.

Opening Cue: Gently stretching back and leg muscles can move you toward a healthier spine.

Cues: The suggestion is to practice 4 breaths as we do strong and steady. You may want to practice long, slow breaths out today.

1. As YOU breathe in, feel the press on the chair... As YOU breathe out, press your hips back any distance. (*Say 4 times slowly.*) When you are ready, come back to standing tall.
2. If you like, do 3 Shoulder Rolls back. As YOU breathe in, shoulders lift... As YOU breathe out, shoulders roll back and down. (*Say 3 times slowly.*)

C. HIP ROCK 'N ROLL

Key Phrase: You can adjust your feet; you are never stuck.

Opening Cue: Gently lifting and tucking the tailbone can help keep spinal discs healthy.

Cues:

1. When you are ready, stand tall with your hands on your hips. Give yourself a moment to tuck your tailbone. Then lift your tailbone. One more time...tuck your tailbone and then lift your tailbone. Notice you can do this motion without moving your legs. This lifting and tucking is hip Rock 'n Roll.
2. When you are ready, gently press shoulders back, hips back, and slightly bend knees. Then get yourself set up again for Kitchen Stretch.
3. Find your own rhythm. As YOU breathe in, lift your tailbone... As YOU breathe out, tuck your tailbone. Take your time as you lift and tuck in hip Rock 'n Roll 3 more times. Always move and breathe in a comfortable way.
4. If you like, next time you lift your tailbone, hold it for 2 breaths. Hold the stretch...but not your breath. Feel the breath in... Feel the breath out. (*Say 2 times slowly.*) Next time you tuck your tailbone, hold it for 2 breaths. Hold the stretch...but not your breath. Feel the breath in... Feel the breath out. (*Say 2 times slowly.*) (**Repeat b.**)

5. Twists (a/c and b/c)

A. GENTLE TWIST: STANDING BEHIND CHAIR (PHOTOS ON P.252)

Key Phrase: You can adjust your stretch anytime; you are never stuck.

Opening Cue: Gentle twists can lengthen the spine and improve circulation.

Cues:

1. We always do both sides. When you are ready, put one hand on the back of the chair. With the other hand, press your palm or a gentle fist on the side of your hip. A different stretch today is to press on the back of your hip bone.
2. Create a comfortable twist as you look to the side.
3. The suggestion is to practice 3 breaths. Find your own rhythm as YOU breathe in, press on your hands... As YOU breathe out, release the press. (*Say 3 times slowly.*) (**Repeat on the other side.**) (**Then do c.**)

B. GENTLE TWIST: FOOT ON CHAIR SEAT (PHOTOS ON P.252)

Key Phrase: We move slowly so you can "find a better way to move."

Opening Cue: The suggestion is to practice one more supported twist to lengthen the spine and improve circulation.

Cues:

1. We always do both sides. When you are ready, put one foot on the seat of the chair. Bring the opposite hand to the side of that leg.
2. Notice if this is a comfortable place to breathe. You can always adjust your twist. Let's take 3 breaths here. Feel the breath in... Feel the breath out. (*Say 3 times slowly.*)
3. Without coming out of the twist, today you may want to look forward or to the other side and create a full spinal twist. Now let's take 3 breaths. Find your own rhythm as YOU breathe in, press on your hands... As YOU breathe out, release the press. (*Say 3 times slowly.*) (**Repeat on the other side.**) (**Then do the Tip-to-Toe Stretch.**)

6. Tip-to-Toe Stretch (photos on p.243)

Opening Cue: (*after a. Gentle Twist: Standing Behind Chair*) Let's do the Tip-to-Toe Stretch again to gently lengthen the spine before we practice another standing twist.

Opening Cue: (*after b. Gentle Twist: Foot on Chair Seat*) Let's practice the Tip-to-Toe Stretch again to gently lengthen the spine before we take a seat.

Cues:

1. When you are ready, stretch one arm to the side or overhead, as we practice the Tip-to-Toe Stretch, fingers stretched wide. Then stretch the other arm to the side or overhead, fingers stretched wide.
2. Find your own rhythm as you stretch from tip-to-toe. Take your time stretching one arm and then the other.
3. When you are ready, arms release.

B. Seated (15 minutes)
1. Get Yourself Set Up

Key Phrases: (1) Anything we do seated, you can do standing or even lying down. (2) You can always find ways to move and to breathe with me.

Opening Cue: Sitting or standing with your shoulders back can take pressure off your back.

Cues:

1. Give yourself a few moments to find a comfortable way to sit today, either on a folded blanket or on a chair.
2. Gently press one shoulder back… Then press the other shoulder back.
3. If you like, move from side to side as you settle into your seat. Perhaps move in a circle. Take your time as you move. You may want to circle even more slowly the other way.
4. Make any adjustments to make your seat more comfortable.

2. The Wave Breath (photos on p.262)

Key Phrases: (1) Long, slow breaths out *can* lower blood pressure. (2) Longer breaths in *can* be energizing.

Opening Cue: You can interrupt your stress cycle by choosing how you breathe.

Cues:

1. Notice if your shoulders are still gently pressed back.
2. The suggestion is to practice 5 breaths as we do the Wave Breath.
   As YOU breathe in, hands lift (*palms up*). As YOU breathe out, release (*palms down*).
   (*Say 2 times slowly.*)
   Always breathe in a comfortable way.
   On YOUR next breath in, hands lift… As YOU breathe out, release.
   As YOU breathe in, hands lift… As YOU breathe out, release.
   (*Say 2 times slowly.*)
3. If you like, gently move the fingers on one hand or shake that hand… Then gently move the fingers on the other hand or shake that hand.

3. Tip-to-Toe Stretch (photos on p.244)

Key Phrase: Different days, different stretches.

Opening Cue: There are many seated stretches that can move you toward a healthier spine.

Cues:

1. When you are ready, stretch one arm to the side or overhead. If you like, stretch your fingers wide. Then stretch the other arm to the side or overhead, fingers stretched wide.

2. Find your own rhythm as you stretch one arm, fingers stretched wide... Then stretch the other arm, fingers spread wide.
3. Take your time with each stretch. Today you may like to stretch your toes as you stretch your fingers wide. When you are ready, arms by your sides.

4. Side-to-Side (Lateral) Stretches (a/b) (photos on p.244)

A. SHOULDER LIFT AND RELEASE

Key Phrase: We move slowly so you can "find a better way to move."

Opening Cue: Bending from side-to-side (lateral stretches) as you sit are two more ways for you to move toward a healthier spine.

Cues: If you like, with your arms by your sides, lift and gently arc one shoulder. Then lift and gently arc the other shoulder. That is 1 set of shoulder lift and release. Find your own rhythm as we do 3 more sets. (*Say 3 times slowly.*)

B. CRESCENT STRETCH

Key Phrase: You can make the stretch as gentle or intense as you need today.

Opening Cue: You may want to continue shoulder lift and release, or today you may want a different stretch.

Cues:

1. We always do both sides. When you are ready, put your hands on your hips. Then, lift or gently arc one shoulder. Today you may want to arc that arm overhead. If you like, stretch your fingers wide. When you are ready, gently lift and arc on the other side. That's 1 set. Find your own rhythm lifting and gently arcing one shoulder or one arm and then the other as you do 2 more sets. Notice if one side feels different than the other. (**Variation.**)
2. The suggestion is now to finish by holding each stretch for 2 breaths. As you lift and gently arc to one side, hold the stretch...but not your breath. Feel the breath in... Feel the breath out. (*Say 2 times slowly.*) When you are ready, lift and gently arc to the other side. If you like, hold the stretch...but not your breath. Feel the breath in... Feel the breath out. (*Say 2 times slowly.*)
3. Now if you like, gently move the fingers on one hand or shake that hand... Then gently move the fingers on the other hand or shake that hand.

Variation: Today you may like to grasp your wrist as you arc one arm overhead. Find your own rhythm as you move from side to side.

5. Cat/Cow (Flex and Extend) (photos on p.242)

Key Phrase: Different days, different stretches.

Opening Cue: Bending forward and back (flexing and extending) the spine as you sit are two more ways you can move toward a healthier spine.

Cues:

1. If you like, tap your *fingertips* on your legs. The suggestion is to practice seated cat/cow 2 times.
2. As YOU breathe in, chin lifts…shoulders back…rock forward.
   As YOU breathe out, chin tucks…shoulders forward…rock back a comfortable distance. Always move and breathe in a comfortable way.
3. On YOUR next breath in, chin lifts…shoulders back…rock forward. As YOU breathe out, chin tucks…shoulders forward…rock back a comfortable distance.
4. When you are ready, come back to sitting tall.

6. Twists and Cat/Cow (a/b)

A. SHOULDER ROCK 'N ROLL (PHOTO ON P.254)

Key Phrase: You can make each stretch as gentle or intense as you need today.

Opening Cue: Gentle seated stretches can release some physical and emotional pain.

Cues:

1. Gently bend your elbows and stretch your fingers if that is comfortable for you today.
2. When you are ready, move one arm across the front, the other arm across the back as we practice shoulder Rock 'n Roll. Leading from the elbows if you like, now move the other arm across the front, and the other across the back. That's 1 set. Find your own rhythm as you practice 2 more sets. You can make each stretch as gentle or intense as you need today. Moving the arms from front to back in any way that feels comfortable… Finding your own rhythm as you move.
3. Now if you like, lead from the shoulders as you move from front to back. Practice as many sets as feels comfortable for you today… Moving the arms from front to back as slowly as you would like.
4. Now, the suggestion is to hold the stretch on each side for 2 breaths. As one shoulder moves across the front and the other across the back, hold

the stretch...but not your breath. Feel the breath in... Feel the breath out. (*Say 2 times slowly.*)
5. Now as your other shoulder moves across the front and the other across the back, hold the stretch...but not your breath. Feel the breath in... Feel the breath out. (*Say 2 times slowly.*)
6. When you are ready, arms to your sides.

B. CLASSIC TWIST WITH CAT/COW (PHOTOS ON P.242)

Key Phrase: There is no place you are trying to go with a stretch.

Opening Cue: The suggestion is to practice one more gentle twist to practice moving toward a healthier spine as you sit.

Cues:

1. Gently press one shoulder back... Then press the other shoulder back. If you like, tap your *fingertips* on your legs.
2. We always do both sides. On YOUR next breath in, press down on hands and feet. As YOU breathe out, bring hands around to one side. (**Variation.**)
3. Let's practice 4 breaths here. As YOU breathe in, hands press. As YOU breathe out, release the press. (*Say 4 times slowly.*)
4. When you are ready, come back to facing front. If you like, tap your *hands* on your legs.
5. Before we do the other side, let's practice 2 cat/cows.
6. As YOU breathe in, chin lifts...shoulders back...rock forward.
7. As YOU breathe out, chin tucks...shoulders forward...rock back a comfortable distance.
   Always move and breathe in a comfortable way.
8. On YOUR next breath in, chin lifts...shoulders back...rock forward. As YOU breathe out, chin tucks...shoulders forward...rock back a comfortable distance.
9. When you are ready, come back to sitting tall. (**Repeat on the other side.**)

Variation: When it feels easy to breathe in the twist, you may want to look forward for a full spinal twist. If you like, practice 4 breaths here.

7. Finger Stretch Breath

Key Phrase: Long, slow breaths out *can* lower heart rate, lower blood pressure, and lower muscle tension.

Opening Cue: One way we can manage pain in real-time is by choosing how we breathe.

Cues: In Finger Stretch Breath, the suggestion is to stretch your fingers about half an inch or a few centimeters. (**Variations.**)

1. When you are ready, gently press one shoulder back... Then press the other shoulder back. If you like, let's practice 5 breaths.
   As YOU breathe in, fingers stretch... As YOU breathe out, release.
   (*Say 2 times slowly.*)
   Always breathe in a comfortable way.
   On YOUR next breath in, fingers stretch... As YOU breathe out, release.
   As YOU breathe in, fingers stretch... As YOU breathe out, release.
   (*Say 2 times slowly.*)
2. If you like, gently move the fingers on one hand or shake that hand... Then gently move the fingers on the other hand or shake that hand.

Variations: (1) Stretch your fingers just enough to notice the stretch. **Or** (2) Stretch your fingers as wide as you would like today. **Or** (3) Perhaps stretch your fingers in a different way today.

C. Lying Down (15 minutes)
1. Get Yourself Set Up (photo on p.258)
Key Phrases: (1) Anything we do lying down, you can do seated or standing. (2) You can always find ways to move and to breathe with me.

Opening Cue: Major muscles that usually work to hold us up can release when we lie down.

Cues: Give yourself a few moments to get yourself set up. You can make adjustments; you are never stuck.

1. You may want a rolled-up blanket, towel, or mat under your knees before you lie back.
2. Today, you may want a small roll (washcloth or towel) under your neck for support.

2. The Noticing Breath
Key Phrase: Long, slow breaths out *can* lower heart rate, lower blood pressure, and lower muscle tension.

Opening Cue: One way we can manage pain in real-time is by choosing how we breathe.

Cues: Notice if you have any area in which you feel discomfort—either physical or emotional. Or pick an area on which to practice—your knee, perhaps.

1. The Noticing Breath is 5 breaths. The suggestion is long, slow breaths out if that is comfortable for you today.
2. When you are ready, gently press one shoulder back... Then press the other shoulder back.
3. On YOUR breath in, notice that area of discomfort... On YOUR breath out, keep noticing. (*Say 2 times slowly.*) Instead of ignoring the discomfort, the suggestion is to keep noticing it as you breathe.
4. On YOUR *next* breath in, notice that area... On YOUR breath out, keep noticing.
   On YOUR breath in, notice that area... On YOUR breath out, keep noticing. (*Say 2 times slowly.*)
5. If you like, gently move the fingers on one hand or shake that hand. Then gently move the fingers on the other hand or shake that hand.
6. You may want to practice the Noticing Breath later, when you want to interrupt your stress cycle.

3. Tip-to-Toe Stretch (photos on p.258)

Key Phrase: Always move in a comfortable way.

Opening Cue: Lying down allows different sets of large muscles to release.

Cues:

1. When you are ready, stretch one arm to the side or overhead as we stretch from tip-to-toe. Then stretch the other arm. Perhaps today add stretching the fingers wide.
2. Find your own rhythm as you move your arms. Take your time with the stretch.
3. When you are ready, press one heel forward and then the other. Keep stretching your arms and pressing your heels forward in any way that feels comfortable for you today. Notice where you feel the stretches as you move.
4. If you like, stretch your fingers and your toes 3 times. As YOU breathe in, fingers and toes stretch...as YOU breathe out, release. (*Say 3 times slowly.*)
5. When you are ready, arms by your sides.

4. Side-to-Side (Lateral) Stretch: Shoulder Lift and Release (photo on p.254)

Key Phrase: You can make each stretch as gentle or intense as you need today.

Opening Cue: We can gently stretch muscles around the neck and shoulders to reduce emotional and physical tension as we are lying down.

Cues: The suggestion is to practice 3 sets of side stretches with your arms by your sides.

1. As YOU breathe in, lift one shoulder toward your ear and press the other shoulder down... As YOU breathe out, lift that shoulder toward your ear and press the other shoulder down. That's 1 set. Keep breathing in a comfortable way as we practice 2 more sets. (*Say 3 times slowly.*)

Variation: When you are ready, arc one arm overhead in a comfortable way; if you like, stretch your fingers wide. Then arc the other arm overhead, fingers stretched wide.

5. Bridge Flow (a/b) (photos on p.259)
A. RAISING YOUR HEART

Key Phrase: Use the pieces of the stretch that feel comfortable for you today.

Opening Cue: When you are lying down, you can release some muscle tension and increase circulation.

Cues: The suggestion is to practice Raising Your Heart 3 times.

1. When you are ready, put your feet on the floor, under your knees.
2. As YOU breathe in, press down on your hips and shoulders, gently raising your heart as you arch your back a comfortable distance.
3. If you like, press your shoulders in toward your spine. Keep breathing in a comfortable way.
4. Notice your next breath in... On YOUR *next* breath out, slowly release, pull your legs in, and wrap your arms around your shins (or backs of your legs). Press as firmly as is comfortable for you today. If you like, we can practice another 2 Raising Your Heart flows. (**Repeat 2 more times.**)

B. BRIDGE LIFT AND RELEASE

Key Phrase: A long, slow breath out can lower heart rate, lower blood pressure, and lower muscle tension.

Opening Cue: Moving in this bridge flow can strengthen core muscles.

Cues: When you are ready, put your feet on the floor under your knees again. The suggestion is to practice bridge lift and release 3 times.

1. As YOU breathe in, press down on your feet and gently lift your hips, any distance. (**Variation.**)
2. On YOUR next breath out, slowly release down and pull your knees in. Perhaps wrap your arms around your shins (or backs of your legs) and press as firmly as is comfortable. (**Repeat 3 times.**)
3. Still in a wrap, if you like, practice 3 breaths. You may want to practice long, slow breaths out. As you breathe in, fingers press... As you breathe out, fingers release. (*Say 2 times slowly.*)

Variation: With your hips still lifted, extend your arms overhead, hands on the floor behind you. If you like, take 2 breaths here. Feel the breath in... Feel the breath out. (*Say 2 times slowly.*)

6. Twists (a/b) (photos on p.000 [AQ])

A. OUTER HIP STRETCH/TWIST

Key Phrase: There is no place you are trying to go with a stretch.

Opening Cue: Gently stretching the outer hip can help keep the spine in better alignment.

Cues:

1. We always do both sides. When you are ready, bend one knee and place that foot above or next to the knee on the other leg.
2. Gently draw that knee across—even a small stretch has benefit. If you like, look the opposite way for a full spinal twist. Notice if this is a comfortable place to breathe. Make any adjustments; you are never stuck.
3. The suggestion is to practice 4 breaths. As YOU breathe in, hands press... As YOU breathe out, release the press. (*Say 4 times slowly.*)

B. SIDE-TO-SIDE ROCKING

Key Phrase: Different days, different stretches.

Opening Cue: Gently moving while lying down can massage connective tissue and reduce muscle tension.

Cues:

1. When you are ready, pull both knees toward you and wrap your hands around fronts of shins or backs of legs.
2. If you like, gently rock from side to side. Today you may want to wiggle your toes.

3. Give yourself a moment to move your feet in any way that feels comfortable. (**Variation.**)
4. Notice your next breath in… As YOU breathe out, release one leg to the floor. Notice your next breath in… As YOU breathe out, release the other leg to the floor. (**Repeat a/b.**)

Variation: Cross your ankles as you rock. If you like, cross your ankles the other way and continue rocking.

7. Anytime, Anywhere Breath

Key Phrase: Long, slow breaths out *can* lower heart rate, lower blood pressure, and lower muscle tension.

Opening Cue: You can interrupt your stress cycle by choosing how you breathe.

Cues: You can do the Anytime, Anywhere Breath even when talking with someone.

1. When you are ready, gently press one shoulder down… Then press the other shoulder down. If you like, place one hand on your leg in a way that is comfortable.
2. The suggestion is to practice long, slow breaths out as we take 5 breaths. (**Variation 1.**)
   As YOU breathe in, fingers press… As YOU breathe out, release.
   (*Say 2 times slowly.*)
   Always breathe in a comfortable way.
   On YOUR next breath in, fingers press… As YOU breathe out, release.
   As YOU breathe in, fingers press… As YOU breathe out, release.
   (*Say 2 times slowly.*)
3. If you like, gently move the fingers on one hand or shake that hand… Then gently move the fingers on the other hand or shake that hand. (**Variation 2.**)
4. You may want to practice the Anytime, Anywhere Breath later when you want to change how you are feeling.

Variations: (1) Press your fingers firmly or gently today. **Or** (2) Now if you like, use your other hand and practice saying it 5 times to yourself in your mind, since *you* are always with you. (*Say slowly during this time so there is no "dead air." Don't rush your words… Don't rush your breath. Take your time with your words… Take your time with your breath.*)

D. FINAL STRETCH (15 MINUTES) (SEE P.218)
1. Get Yourself Set Up (photo on p.258)

2. Final Stretch: A Body-Based, Guided Meditation

E. Make a Plan

F. Extras
1. Time Adjustments
Running Out of Time? After lying down side-to-side (lateral) stretch, go to side-to-side rocking and then Final Stretch.

2. Theme Variation: Savor the Stretch
After you have done this practice several times, you can offer this idea at the beginning and mention it a few times during the practice:

> Today, you might want to move even more slowly than in our last practice. Give yourself a moment to Savor the Stretch.

3. Ideas to extend to a 90-minute practice
A. * SUPPORTED BACKBEND (PHOTOS ON P.246)
Key Phrase: Only move in a comfortable way.

Opening Cue: Let's practice two more stretches to move the spine forward and back.

Cues:

1. When you are ready, stand with your knees slightly bent. Place your palms or gentle fists on your hips or on the middle of your hip bone in the back.
2. The suggestion is to keep your chin level as you press your shoulders and elbows back to create a comfortable supported backbend. If you like, take 3 breaths. Feel the breath in... Feel the breath out. (*Say 3 times slowly.*)
3. When you are ready, come back to standing tall. Notice the gentle bend in your knees.
4. If you like, press your shoulders forward and tuck your chin and take 2 breaths here. Feel the breath in... Feel the breath out. (*Say 2 times slowly.*)
5. Let's do that one more time. (**Repeat entire stretch.**)
6. When you are ready, hands by your sides. If you like, gently move the fingers on one hand or shake that hand... Then gently move the fingers on the other hand or shake that hand.

B. * CRESCENT STRETCH VARIATION (PHOTOS ON P.245)

Key Phrase: Make the stretch as gentle or intense as you need today.

Opening Cue: Moving slowly allows us "to find a better way to move."

Cues:

1. We always do both sides. When you are ready, arc one arm and grasp that wrist as you create a crescent stretch. Stretch your fingers wide. **(Repeat on the other side.)**
2. If you like, hold each stretch for 2 breaths. On one side, hold the stretch… but not your breath. Feel the breath in… Feel the breath out. (*Say 2 times slowly.*) When you are ready, on the other side, hold the stretch…but not your breath. Feel the breath in… Feel the breath out. (*Say 2 times slowly.*)

C. * 1-2-3 SHOULDER STRETCH VARIATION

Key Phrase: Even small stretches have benefits.

Opening Cue: Let's continue to move the spine forward and back as we sit.

Cues:

1. The suggestion is to bend your elbows if that is comfortable for you today as we do the 1-2-3 Shoulder Stretch Variation.
2. As YOU breathe in, press both shoulders back and lift your chin a comfortable distance. That's 1. As YOU breathe out, press both shoulders forward and tuck the chin. That's 2.
   When you are ready, release the stretch. That's 3.
3. You can make each stretch as gentle or intense as you need today. If you like, let's practice this stretch 2 more times. (*Say slowly 2 more times.*)

D. EXTENDED MAKE A PLAN (P.220)

PART IV
APPENDICES

APPENDIX A

Practice Sequence Photographs

Many thanks to our yoga model, Elizabeth Q. Finlinson, LCSW

TREE POSE

Side 1   Side 2

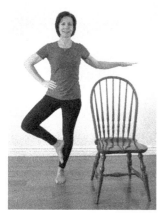
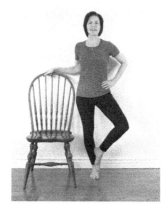
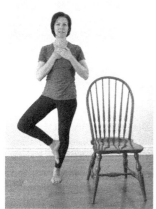
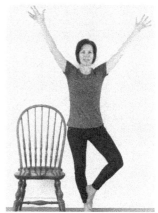
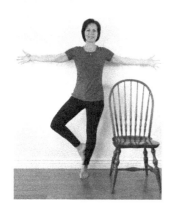
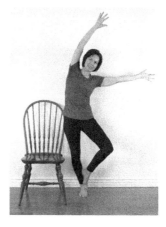

EAGLE POSE

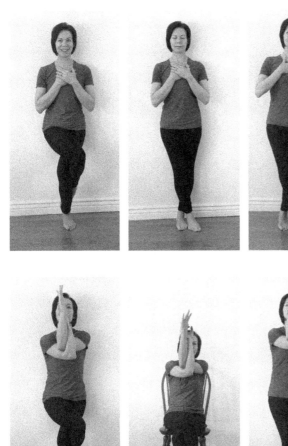
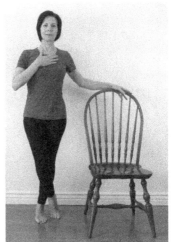
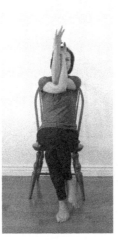
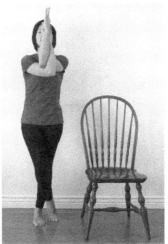

TAKE UP SPACE

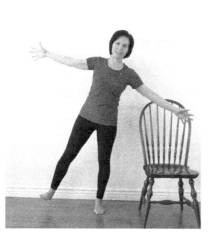
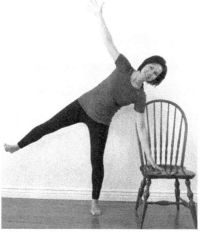

SEATED TWIST WITH CAT/COW

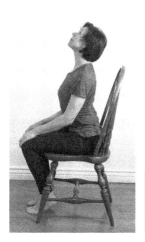
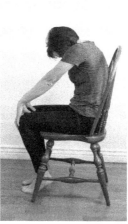
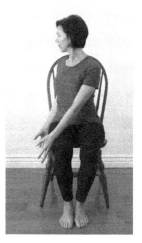

TIP-TO-TOE

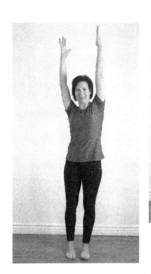
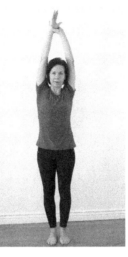
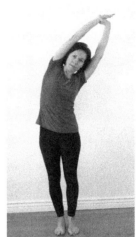
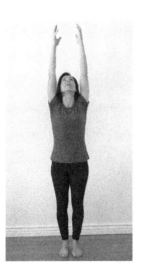
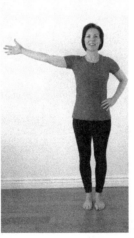
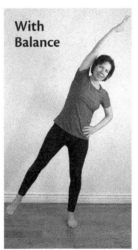

With Balance

SEATED TIP-TO-TOE

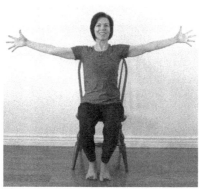

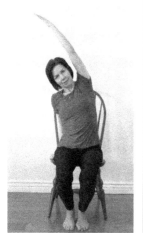 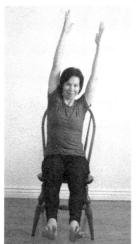 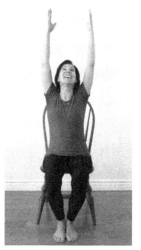

Seated Side-to-Side Stretches

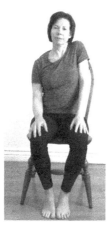 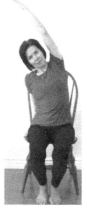

WIDE-LEGGED ADD-ON

Edges of Feet

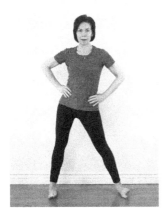

Hips to Side

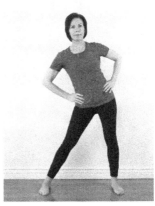

Shoulder Arc

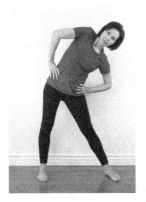

Crescent

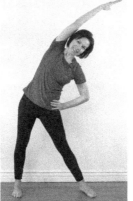

With Balance

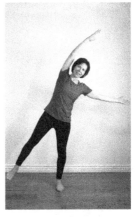

WARRIOR 1 FLOW

Achilles Stretch

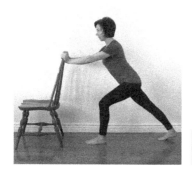 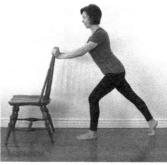

Warrior 1

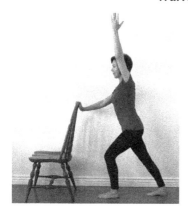 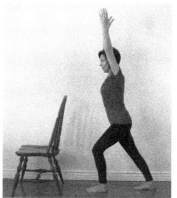

Supported Backbend

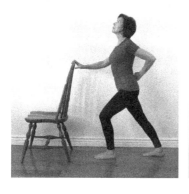 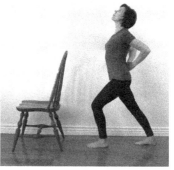

WARRIOR 1 FLOW

Twists

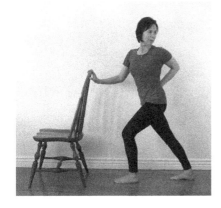
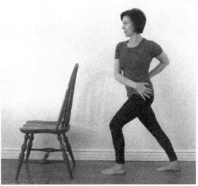

Core Check

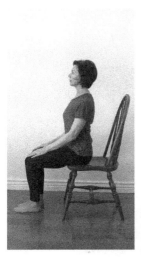
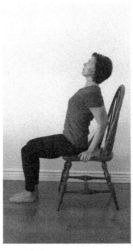
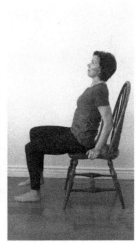

CORE CHECK

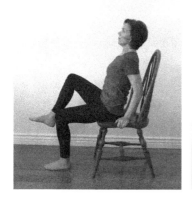
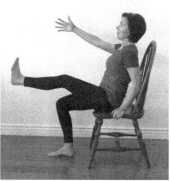
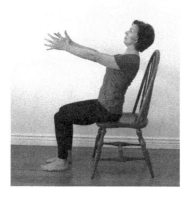
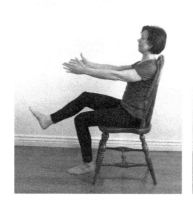
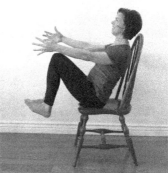

RING THE BELL

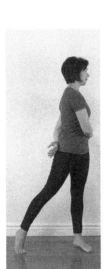
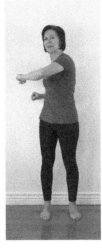
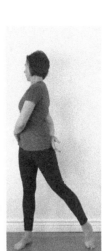
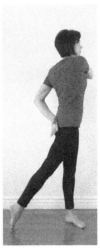

KITCHEN STRETCH
Set Up

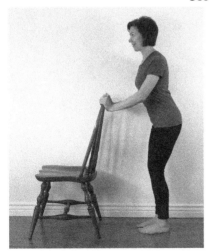
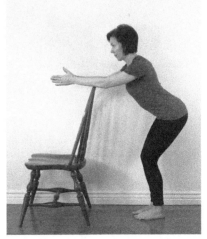

KITCHEN STRETCH

| Strong & Steady | Hamstring Stretch |

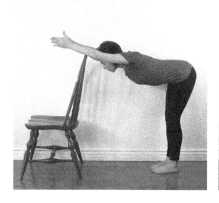
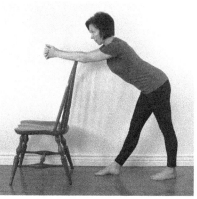

Hip Rock 'n Roll (lift)

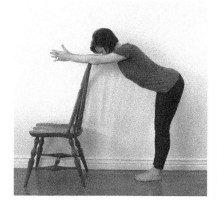
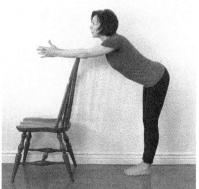

Psoas & Glute Stretch

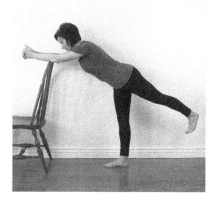
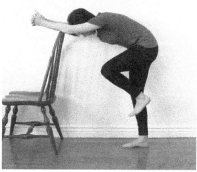

LYING DOWN #4 STRETCHES

Hip Stretch **Hamstring Stretch**

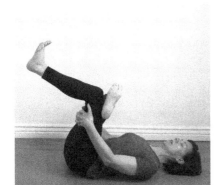 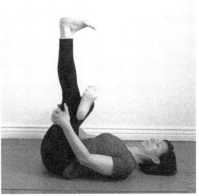

SEATED #4 STRETCHES

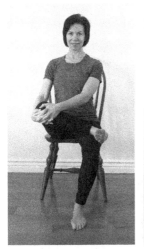 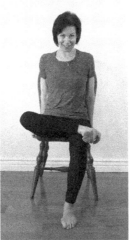 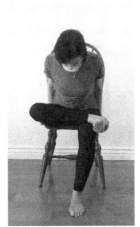

STANDING #4 STRETCH

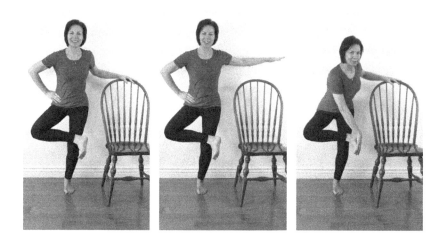

TWISTS

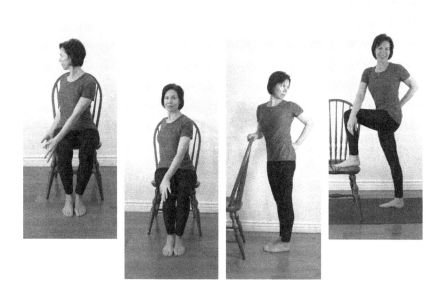

HIP & CORE STRENGTHENING

Pendulum

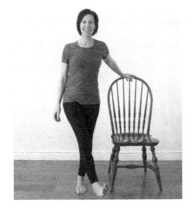
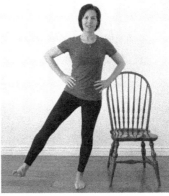

Warrior 3 Flow

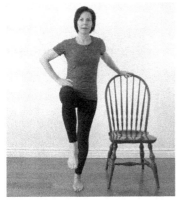
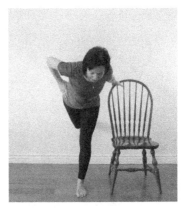

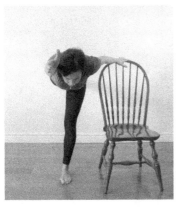
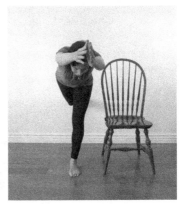

THE SHOULDER SUITE

Lift & Release　　　Forward & Back　　　Shoulder Rock 'n Roll

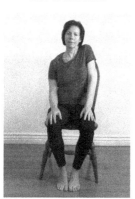 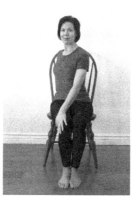 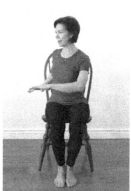

1-2-3 STRETCH

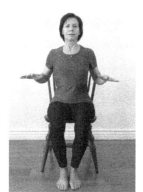 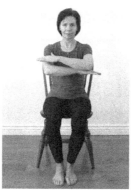 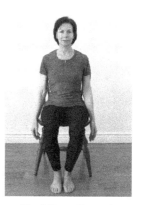

Shoulder Rolls　　　　　　　Find Own Stretch

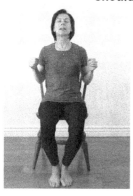 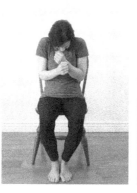 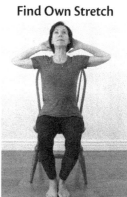

NECK & SHOULDER SUITE

Neck Massage
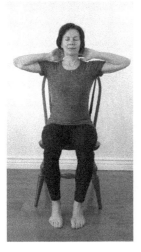

Chin Lift & Release
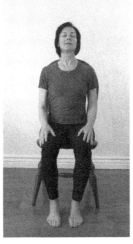

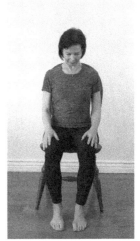

Pendulum
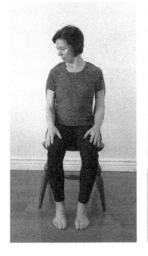

Head Tilt
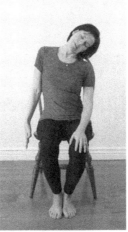

Shoulder Roll
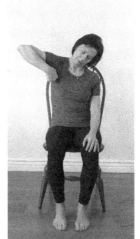

KNEEL 'N STRETCH

Set Up | Hip Rock 'n Roll

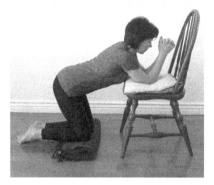 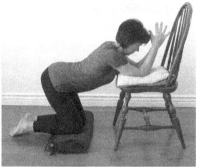

Extend & Tuck

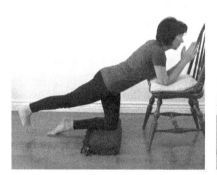 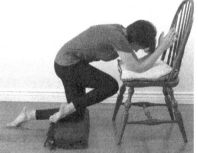

Twist

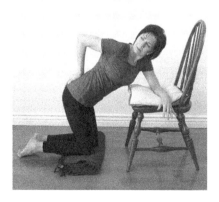

QUAD & PSOAS STRETCHES

Quad Stretch	Psoas Stretch

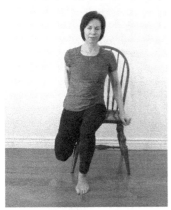
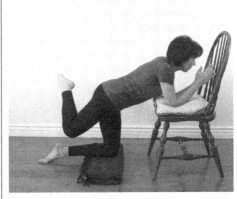
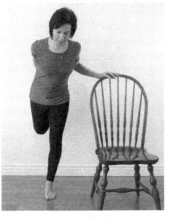
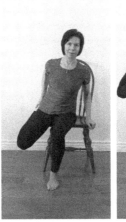
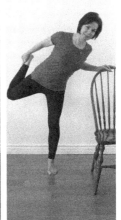
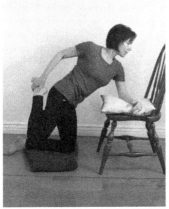

GET YOURSELF SET UP

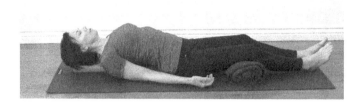

LYING DOWN TIP-TO-TOE

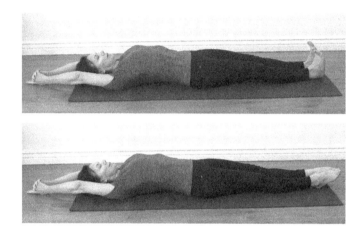

GENTLE TWIST WITH KNEES

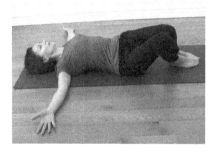
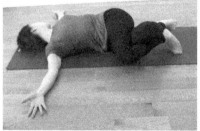

RAISING YOUR HEART

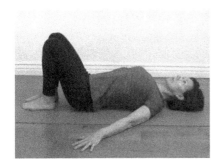 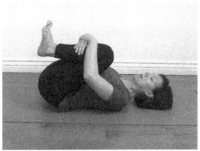

BRIDGE LIFT & RELEASE

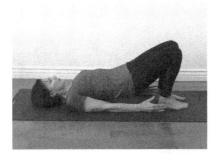 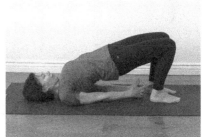

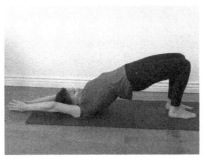 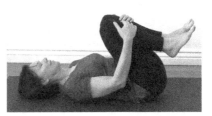

Back Release	Spiral Knees
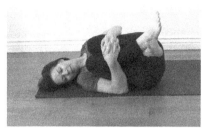	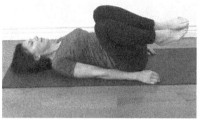

SEATED HIP TO TOE

Footwork	Knee	Hip
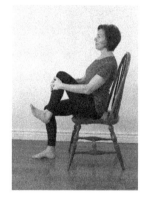	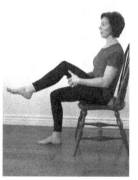	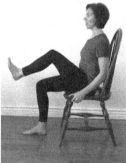

HIP TO TOE STRETCHES

Toes/Foot/Ankle

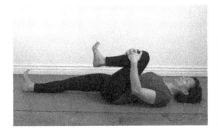

Spiral Knees

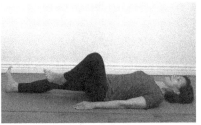

Knee Stretch

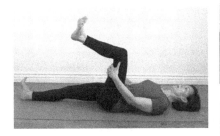

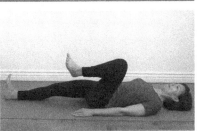

Outer Hip/Twist

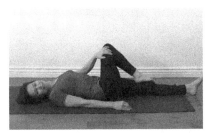

BREATHWORK

Gently Move Fingers, Gently Shake Hand

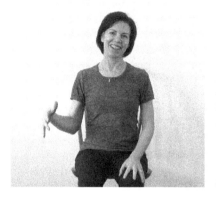

Feel the Breath

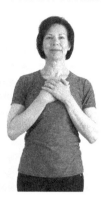

The Wave Breath

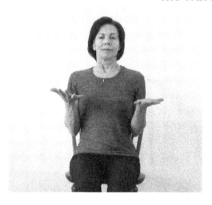
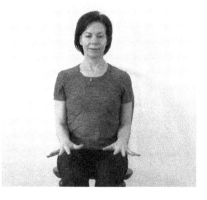

Finger Stretch Breath & The Physiological Sigh

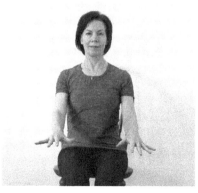

Anytime, Anywhere Breath

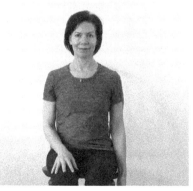

APPENDIX B

Resources

These resources have shaped the GreenTREE Yoga® Approach.

Books and audio books
Breathing
Kahn, S. and Erlich, P. (2018) *Jaws: The Story of a Hidden Epidemic.* Stanford, CA: Stanford University Press.
Nestor, J. (2020) *Breath: The New Science of a Lost Art.* New York: Riverhead Books.

Mindfulness
Bell, C. (2016) *Mindful Yoga, Mindful Life: A Guide for Everyday Practice.* Boulder, CO: Shambhala Press.
Kornfield, J. (2008) *The Wise Heart: A Guide to the Universal Teachings of Buddhist Psychology.* London: Bantam Press.

Movement
Bell, C. (2018) *Hip-Healthy Asana: The Yoga Practitioner's Guide to Protecting the Hips and Avoiding SI Joint Pain.* Boulder, CO: Shambhala Press.
Feldenkrais, M. (reprint 2019) *Awareness Through Movement: Easy-to-Do Health Exercises to Improve Your Posture, Vision, Imagination, and Personal Awareness.* San Francisco, CA: HarperOne.
Feldenkrais, M. (1981/2019) *The Elusive Obvious: The Convergence of Movement, Neuroplasticity & Health.* Berkeley, CA: North Atlantic Press.
Ratey, J. (2013/2018) *Spark: The Revolutionary New Science of Exercise and the Brain.* Boston, MA: Little, Brown & Co.

Neuroscience/Neuroplasticity
Doidge, N. (2015) *The Brain's Way of Healing: Remarkable Discoveries and Recoveries from the Frontiers of Neuroplasticity.* London: Penguin Life.
Eagleman, D. (2020) *Livewired: The Inside Story of the Ever-Changing Brain.* New York: Random House.
Merzenich, M. (2013) *Soft-Wired: How the New Science of Brain Plasticity Can Change Your Life.* San Francisco, CA: Parnassus Publishing.
Porges, S. (2017) *The Pocket Guide to the Polyvagal Theory: The Transformative Power of Feeling Safe.* New York: W.W. Norton & Co.

Porges, S. (2021) *Polyvagal Safety: Attachment, Communication, Self-Regulation*. New York: W.W. Norton & Co.

Siegel, D. (2020) *The Developing Mind: How Relationships and the Brain Interact to Shape Who We Are* (3rd edn). New York: Guilford Press.

Pain Management and Yoga

Levine, P. (2012) *Freedom from Pain*. Louisville, CO: Sounds True.

Pearson, N., Prosko, S., and Sullivan, M. (2019) *Yoga and Science in Pain Care: Treating the Person in Pain*. London and Philadelphia, PA: Singing Dragon.

Trauma

Calhoun, Y. (2024) *Building Safety with Trauma-Informed Yoga: A Practical Guide for Teachers and Clinicians.* New York: Routledge.

Levine, P. (2015) *Trauma and Memory: Brain and Body in a Search for the Living Past*. Berkeley, CA: North Atlantic Press.

Ogden, P. (2006) *Trauma and the Body: A Sensorimotor Approach to Psychotherapy*. New York: W.W. Norton & Co.

Prison Yoga Project (no date) *Yoga: A Path for Healing and Recovery*; *Freedom from the Inside: A Woman's Yoga Practice Guide*. www.prisonyoga.org [books for incarcerated people]

van der Kolk, B. (2015) *The Body Keeps the Score: Brain, Mind, and Body in the Healing of Trauma*. London: Penguin Publishing.

Podcasts

Huberman Lab, podcast episodes (https://hubermanlab.com/category/podcast-episodes):

- How to Breathe Correctly for Optimal Health, Mood, Learning & Performance: https://hubermanlab.com/how-to-breathe-correctly-for-optimal-health-mood-learning-and-performance

- Master Stress: Tools for Managing Stress & Anxiety: https://hubermanlab.com/tools-for-managing-stress-and-anxiety

- Control Pain & Health Faster with Your Brain: https://hubermanlab.com/control-pain-and-heal-faster-with-your-brain

- Master Your Breathing with Dr. Jack Feldman, Breathing for Mental & Physical Health & Performance: https://hubermanlab.com/dr-jack-feldman-breathing-for-mental-physical-health-and-performance

Author Bios

Yael Calhoun, MA, MS, E-RYT, is a long-time educator and author/series editor of over 20 books and manuals. Yael is the Executive Director of GreenTREE Yoga®, a nonprofit dedicated to bringing the benefits of yoga to underserved populations and to those who work with them. Books include: *Building Safety with Trauma-Informed Yoga: A Practical Guide for Teachers and Clinicians* (Routledge Press, 2024) and *Art and Yoga for Children with Differing Needs and Autism: Improve Body Awareness, Sensory Integration and Emotional Regulation* (Singing Dragon, 2025).

Mona Bingham, PhD, RN, retired after obtaining the rank of Colonel, serving as Consultant to the Surgeon General for Nursing Research and Chief of Nursing Research at Brooke Army Medical Center. Her research interest in integrative medicine (primarily pain, sleep, and other post-traumatic stress disorder (PTSD) issues post deployment) began after she returned from her 2003 deployment for Operation Enduring Freedom and Operation Iraqi Freedom (OEF/OIF). She has continued her research and consulting, and has attended Yael's classes for years.

Endnotes

Introduction

1. See www.iasp-pain.org/publications/iasp-news/iasp-announces-revised-definition-of-pain

Chapter 1

1. Fisher, J.P., Hassan, D.T., and O'Connor, N. (1995) "Minerva." *British Medical Journal 310*, 70. https://doi.org/10.1136/bmj.310.6971.70
2. von Bartheld, C.S., Bahney, J., and Herculano-Houzel, S. (2016) "The search for true numbers of neurons and glial cells in the human brain: A review of 150 years of cell counting." *The Journal of Comparative Neurology 524*, 18, 3865–3895. doi: 10.1002/cne.24040.
3. Doidge, N. (2007) *The Brain that Changes Itself: Stories of Personal Triumph from the Frontiers of Brain Science*. London: Penguin Books.
4. Eagleman, D. (2020) *Livewired: The Inside Story of the Ever-Changing Brain*. New York: Random House.
5. Hebb, D.O. (1952) *The Organization of Behavior: Neuropsychological Theory*. New York: John Wiley & Sons.
6. Carla Shatz, quoted in Collins, N. (2017) "Pathways: From the eye to the brain." *Stanford Medicine Magazine*, August 21. https://biox.stanford.edu/highlight/pathways-eye-brain
7. Doidge, N. (2007) *The Brain's Way of Healing: Stories of Remarkable Recoveries and Discoveries*. London: Allen Lane.
8. Fishman, L. and Ardman, C. (2012) *Yoga for Back Pain*. New York: W.W. Norton & Co.
9. Finnerup, N.B., Haroutounian, S., Kamerman, P., Baron, R., et al. (2016) "Neuropathic pain: An updated grading system for research and clinical practice." *Pain 157*, 8, 1599–1606. doi: 10.1097/j.pain.0000000000000492.
10. Song, K.-S., Cho, J.H., Hong, J.-Y., Lee, J.H., et al. (2017) "Neuropathic pain related with spinal disorders: A systematic review." *Asian Spine Journal 11*, 4, 661–674. doi: 10.4184/asj.2017.11.4.661.
11. Harvard Medical School (2016) *Neck Pain: A Troubleshooting Guide to Help You Relieve Your Pain, Restore Function, and Prevent Injury*. Special Health Reports. Boston, MA: Harvard Medical School, Harvard Health Publishing, www.health.harvard.edu/pain/neck-pain-a-troubleshooting-guide-to-help-you-relieve-your-pain-restore-function-and-prevent-injury, p.14.
12. Alshelh, Z., Di Pietro, F., Youssef, A.M., Reeves, J.M., et al. (2016) "Chronic neuropathic pain: It's about the rhythm." *The Journal of Neuroscience 36*, 3, 1008–1018. www.jneurosci.org/content/36/3/1008
13. Donnelly, C.R., Andriessen, A.S., Chen, G., Wang, K., et al. (2020) "Central nervous system targets: Glial cell mechanisms in chronic pain." *Neurotherapeutics 17*, 3, 846–860. doi: 10.1007/s13311-020-00905-7.
14. R. Douglas Fields, quoted in Dobbs, D. (2021) "The quiet scientific revolution that may solve chronic pain." *The New York Times*, November 9, www.nytimes.com/2021/11/09/well/mind/glial-cells-chronic-pain-treatment.html?smid=url-share
15. Elliot Krane, quoted in Dobbs, D. (2021) "The quiet scientific revolution that may solve chronic pain." *The New York Times*, November 9, www.nytimes.com/2021/11/09/well/mind/glial-cells-chronic-pain-treatment.html?smid=url-share

16. Ramachandran, V.S. (2012) *The Tell-Tale Brain: A Neuroscientist's Quest for What Makes Us Human.* New York: W.W. Norton & Co.
17. Saadon-Grosman, N., Loewenstein, Y., and Arzy, S. (2020) "The 'creatures' of the human cortical somatosensory system." *Brain Communications* 2, 1, 1-10.
18. Pearson, N., Prosko, S., and Sullivan, M. (2019) *Yoga and Science in Pain Care: Treating the Person in Pain.* London and Philadelphia, PA: Singing Dragon, Chapter 5.
19. US Department of Health and Human Services (2019) *Pain Management Best Practices Inter-Agency Task Force Report: Updates, Gaps, Inconsistencies, and Recommendations. Final Report.* US Department of Health and Human Services, US Department of Defense, US Department of Veterans Affairs, and Office of National Drug Control Policy, May. www.hhs.gov/sites/default/files/pmtf-final-report-2019-05-23.pdf
20. Sean Mackey, quoted in Sutherland, S. (2017) "Rethinking relief." *Scientific American Mind* 28, 3, 28-35. doi: 10.1038/scientificamericanmind0517-28.

Chapter 2

1. Lieberman, D.E. (2020) *Exercised: Why Something We Never Evolved to Do Is Healthy and Rewarding.* Boston, MA: Harvard University.
2. Ratey, J., with Hagerman, E. (2008 [2013]) *Spark: The Revolutionary New Science of Exercise and the Brain.* Boston, MA: Little, Brown & Co.
3. Page, P. (2012) "Current concepts in muscle stretching for exercise and rehabilitation." *International Journal of Sports Physical Therapy* 7, 1, 109-119.
4. Fishman, L. and Ardman, C. (2012) *Yoga for Back Pain.* New York: W.W. Norton & Co, p.16.
5. Häkkinen, A., Kautiainen, H., Hannonen, P., and Ylinen, J. (2008) "Strength training and stretching versus stretching only in the treatment of patients with chronic neck pain: A randomized one-year follow-up study." *Clinical Rehabilitation* 22, 7, 592-600. doi: 10.1177/0269215507087486.
6. Ylinen, J., Kautiainen, H., Wirén, K., and Häkkinen, A. (2007) "Stretching exercises vs manual therapy in treatment of chronic neck pain: A randomized, controlled cross-over trial." *Journal of Rehabilitation Medicine* 39, 2, 126-132. doi: 10.2340/16501977-0015.
7. da Cruz Fernandes, I., Pinto, R.Z., Ferreira, P., and Lira, F.S. (2018) "Low back pain, obesity, and inflammatory markers: Exercise as potential treatment." *Journal of Exercise Rehabilitation* 14, 2, 168-174. doi: 10.12965/jer.1836070.035.
8. Belavy, D.L., Van Oosterwijck, J., Clarkson, M., Dhondt, E., et al. (2021) "Pain sensitivity is reduced by exercise training: Evidence from a systematic review and meta-analysis." *Neuroscience & Biobehavioral Reviews* 120, 100-108. doi: 10.1016/j.neubiorev.2020.11.012.
9. Pacheco-Barrios, K., Gianiorenco, A., Machado, R., and Queiroga, M. (2020) "Exercise-induced pain threshold modulation in healthy subjects: A systematic review and meta-analysis." *Principles and Practice of Clinical Research Journal* 6, 3, 11-28. doi: 10.21801/ppcrj.2020.63.2.
10. Berrueta, L., Muskaj, I., Olenich, S., Butler, T., et al. (2016) "Stretching impacts inflammation resolution in connective tissue." *Journal of Cellular Physiology* 231, 7, 1621-1627. doi: 10.1002/jcp.25263.
11. Lieberman, D.E. (2020) *Exercised: Why Something We Never Evolved to Do Is Healthy and Rewarding.* Boston, MA: Harvard University, p.64.
12. Emery, C.F., Kiecolt-Glaser, J.K., Glaser, R., Malarkey, W.B., and Frid, D.J. (2005) "Exercise accelerates wound healing among healthy older adults: A preliminary investigation." *The Journals of Gerontology. Series A, Biological Sciences and Medical Sciences* 60, 11, 1432-1436. doi: 10.1093/gerona/60.11.1432.
13. Sarno, J.E. (1998) *The Mindbody Prescription: Healing the Body, Healing the Pain.* New York: Warner Books Inc.
14. Fishman, L. and Ardman, C. (2012) *Yoga for Back Pain.* New York: W.W. Norton & Co., p.52.
15. Lieberman, D.E. (2020) *Exercised: Why Something We Never Evolved to Do Is Healthy and Rewarding.* Boston, MA: Harvard University, p.268.
16. Basso, J.C. and Suzuki, W.A. (2017) "The effects of acute exercise on mood, cognition, neurophysiology, and neurochemical pathways: A review." *Brain Plasticity (Amsterdam, Netherlands)* 2, 2, 127-152. doi: 10.3233/BPL-160040.

17 Young, S.N. (2007) "How to increase serotonin in the human brain without drugs." *Journal of Psychiatry & Neuroscience 32*, 6, 394–399.
18 Wang, J., Liu, S., Li, G., and Xiao, J. (2020) "Exercise regulates the immune system." *Advances in Experimental Medicine and Biology 1228*, 395–408. doi: 10.1007/978-981-15-1792-1_27.
19 Feldenkrais, M. (1972/1977/1990) *Awareness Through Movement: Health Exercises for Personal Growth*. San Francisco, CA: HarperOne, pp.36–37.
20 Birbaumer, N. (2006) "Breaking the silence: Brain–computer interfaces (BCI) for communication and motor control." *Psychophysiology 43*, 6, 517–532. doi: 10.1111/j.1469-8986.2006.00456.x.
21 Camargo-Vargas, D., Callejas-Cuervo, M., and Mazzoleni, S. (2021) "Brain–computer interfaces systems for upper and lower limb rehabilitation: A systematic review." *Sensors 21*, 13, 4312. https://doi.org/10.3390/s21134312
22 Stifani, N. (2014) "Motor neurons and the generation of spinal motor neuron diversity." *Frontiers in Cellular Neuroscience 8*, 293. https://doi.org/10.3389/fncel.2014.00293
23 Harvard Medical School (2020) *Core Exercises: 6 Workouts to Tighten Your Abs, Strengthen Your Back, and Improve Balance*. Special Health Report. Boston, MA: Harvard Health Publishing. www.health.harvard.edu/exercise-and-fitness/core-exercises-6-workouts-to-tighten-your-abs-strengthen-your-back-and-improve-balance, p.6.
24 Feldenkrais, M. (1981/2019) *The Elusive Obvious: The Convergence of Movement, Neuroplasticity & Health*. Berkeley, CA: North Atlantic Books, p.92.
25 Anderson, R. (1980/2020) *Stretching*. Bolinas, CA: Shelter Publications.
26 Fishman, L. and Ardman, C. (2012) *Yoga for Back Pain*. New York: W.W. Norton & Co., p.55.
27 Wyon, M., Felton, L., and Galloway, S. (2009) "A comparison of two stretching modalities on lower-limb range of motion measurements in recreational dancers." *Journal of Strength and Conditioning Research 23*, 7, 2144–2148. doi: 10.1519/JSC.0b013e3181b3e198.
28 Wyon, M., Felton, L., and Galloway, S. (2009) "A comparison of two stretching modalities on lower-limb range of motion measurements in recreational dancers." *Journal of Strength and Conditioning Research 23*, 7, 2144–2148. doi: 10.1519/JSC.0b013e3181b3e198.
29 Bandy, W.D., Irion, J.M., and Briggler, M. (1997) "The effect of time and frequency of static stretching on flexibility of the hamstring muscles." *Physical Therapy 77*, 10, 1090–1096. https://doi.org/10.1093/ptj/77.10.1090
30 Ayala, F. and Sainz de Baranda Andújar, P. (2010) "Effect of 3 different active stretch durations on hip flexion range of motion." *Journal of Strength and Conditioning Research 24*, 2, 430–436. doi: 10.1519/JSC.0b013e3181c0674f.
31 Cipriani, D., Abel, B., and Pirrwitz, D. (2003) "A comparison of two stretching protocols on hip range of motion: Implications for total daily stretch duration." *Journal of Strength and Conditioning Research 17*, 2, 274–278. doi: 10.1519/1533-4287(2003)017<0274:acotsp>2.0.co;2.
32 da Costa, B.R. and Vieira, E.R. (2008) "Stretching to reduce work-related musculoskeletal disorders: A systematic review." *Journal of Rehabilitation Medicine 40*, 5, 321–328. doi: 10.2340/16501977-0204.
33 Hlaing, S.S., Puntumetakul, R., Khine, E.E., and Boucaut, R. (2021) "Effects of core stabilization exercise and strengthening exercise on proprioception, balance, muscle thickness and pain related outcomes in patients with subacute nonspecific low back pain: A randomized controlled trial." *BMC Musculoskeletal Disorders 22*, 99. https://bmcmusculoskeletdisord.biomedcentral.com/articles/10.1186/s12891-021-04858-6
34 Akhtar, M.W., Karimi, H., and Gilani, S.A. (2017) "Effectiveness of core stabilization exercises and routine exercise therapy in management of pain in chronic non-specific low back pain: A randomized controlled clinical trial." *Pakistan Journal of Medical Science 33*, 4, 1002–1006. doi: 10.12669/pjms.334.12664.
35 Chang, W.-D., Lin, H.-Y., and Lai, P.-T. (2015) "Core strength training for patients with chronic low back pain." *Journal of Physical Therapy Science 27*, 3, 619–622. doi: 10.1589/jpts.27.619.

Chapter 3

1. Siegel, D. (2012/2020/2022) *The Developing Mind: How Relationships and the Brain Interact to Shape Who We Are*. New York: Guilford Press, p.2.
2. MacLean, P. (1990) *The Triune Brain in Evolution: Role in Paleocerebral Functions*. New York: Plenum.
3. Kahneman, D. (2011) *Thinking Fast and Slow*. New York: Farrar, Straus, & Giroux, pp.21–22.
4. Ledoux, J. (2015) *Anxious: Using the Brain to Understand Fear and Anxiety*. New York: Viking Press, p.210.
5. Melzack, R. and Wall, P.D. (1965) "Pain mechanisms: A new theory." *Science 150*, 3699, 971–979. doi: 10.1126/science.150.3699.971.
6. Sapolsky, R. (2017) *Behave: The Biology of Humans at Our Best and Worst*. London: Penguin Press, p.699.
7. Patrick Wall, quoted in Mendell, L.M. (2014) "Constructing and deconstructing the gate theory of pain." *Pain 155*, 2, 210–216.
8. Purves, D. and Williams, S.M. (2001) *Neuroscience* (2nd edn). Sunderland, MA: Sinauer Associates, p.8.
9. Pearson, N., Prosko, S., and Sullivan, M. (2019) *Yoga and Science in Pain Care: Treating the Person in Pain*. London and Philadelphia, PA: Singing Dragon, pp.102–103.
10. Harvard Medical School (2016) *Back Pain: Finding Solutions for Your Aching Back*. Special Health Reports. Boston, MA: Harvard Health Publishing, www.health.harvard.edu/pain/back-pain-finding-solutions-for-your-aching-back
11. Vinstrup, J., Jakobsen, M.D., and Andersen, L.L. (2020) "Perceived stress and low-back pain among healthcare workers: A multi-center prospective cohort study." *Frontiers in Public Health 8*, 297. doi: 10.3389/fpubh.2020.00297.
12. Sapolsky, R. (2017) *Behave: The Biology of Humans at Our Best and Worst*. London: Penguin Press, p.41.
13. Stanley, E. (2019) *Widen the Window: Training Your Brain and Body to Thrive During Stress and Recover from Trauma*. New York: Avery, p.315.
14. Ashar, Y.K., Gordon, A., and Schubiner, H. (2022) "Effect of pain reprocessing therapy vs. placebo and usual care for patients with chronic back pain: A randomized clinical trial." *JAMA Psychiatry 79*, 1, 13–23. doi:10.1001/jamapsychiatry.2021.2669
15. Cherkin, D.C., Sherman, K.J., Balderson, B.H., Cook, A.J., et al. (2016) "Effect of mindfulness-based stress reduction vs. cognitive behavioral therapy or usual care on back pain and functional limitations in adults with chronic low back pain: A randomized clinical trial." *JAMA 315*, 12, 1240–1249. doi: 10.1001/jama.2016.2323.
16. Kabat-Zinn, J. (1995/2005) *Wherever You Go, There You Are*. London: Hachette Books, p.15.
17. Foster, N.E., Anema, J.R., Cherkin, D., Chou, R., et al. (2018) "Prevention and treatment of low back pain: Evidence, challenges, and promising directions." *The Lancet 391*, 10137, 2368–2383. doi: 10.1016/S0140-6736(18)30489-6.
18. Bodes Pardo, G., Girbés, E.L., Roussel, N.A., Izquierdo, T.G., Penick, V.J., and Martín, D.P. (2018) "Pain neurophysiology education and therapeutic exercise for patients with chronic low back pain." *Archives of Physical Medicine and Rehabilitation 99*, 2, 338–347. doi: 10.1016/j.apmr.2017.10.016.
19. Zahari, Z., Ishak, A., and Justine, M. (2020) "The effectiveness of patient education in improving pain, disability, and quality of life among older people with low back pain: A systematic review." *Journal of Back and Musculoskeletal Rehabilitation 33*, 2, 245–254. doi: 10.3233/bmr-181305.
20. Puentedura, E.J. and Flynn, T. (2016) "Combining manual therapy with pain neuroscience education in the treatment of chronic low back pain: A narrative review of the literature." *Physiotherapy Theory and Practice 32*, 5, 408–414. doi: 10.1080/09593985.2016.1194663.
21. Pearson, N., Prosko, S., and Sullivan, M. (2019) *Yoga and Science in Pain Care: Treating the Person in Pain*. London and Philadelphia, PA: Singing Dragon, p.103.
22. Porges, S. (2017) *Polyvagal Theory: Neurophysiological Foundations of Emotions, Attachment, Communication, and Self-Regulation*. New York: W.W. Norton & Co.
23. Kornfield, J. (2009) *The Wise Heart: A Guide to the Universal Teachings of Buddhist Psychology*. London: Bantam Press, Chapter 7.
24. Nestor, J. (2020) *Breath: The New Science of a Lost Art*. New York: Riverhead Books.
25. Del Negro, C.A., Funk, G.D., and Feldman, J.L. (2018) "Breathing matters." *Nature Reviews. Neuroscience 19*, 6, 351–367. doi: 10.1038/s41583-018-0003-6.

26　Del Negro, C.A., Funk, G.D., and Feldman, J.L. (2018) "Breathing matters." *Nature Reviews. Neuroscience 19*, 6, 351–367. doi: 10.1038/s41583-018-0003-6.
27　Huberman, A. (2023) "How to Breathe Correctly for Optimal Health" [YouTube video]. https://hubermanlab.com/how-to-breathe-correctly-for-optimal-health-mood-learning-and-performance
28　Smith, J.C., Ellenberger, H.H., Ballanyi, K., Richter, D.W., and Feldman, J.L. (1991) "Pre-Bötzinger complex: A brainstem region that may generate respiratory rhythm in mammals." *Science 254*, 5032, 726–729. doi: 10.1126/science.1683005.
29　Balestrino, M. and Somjen, G.G. (1988) "Concentration of carbon dioxide, interstitial pH and synaptic transmission in hippocampal formation of the rat." *The Journal of Physiology 396*, 1, 247–266. https://doi.org/10.1113/jphysiol.1988.sp016961
30　See https://hubermanlab.com/how-to-breathe-correctly-for-optimal-health-mood-learning-and-performance
31　Porges, S.W. (1995) "Orienting in a defensive world: Mammalian modifications of our evolutionary heritage. A Polyvagal Theory." *Psychophysiology 32*, 4, 301–318. doi: 10.1111/j.1469-8986.1995.tb01213.x.
32　Porges, S. (2017) *Polyvagal Theory: Neurophysiological Foundations of Emotions, Attachment, Communication, and Self-Regulation*. New York: W.W. Norton & Co., pp.191–192.
33　Basso, J.C. and Suzuki, W.A. (2017) "The effects of acute exercise on mood, cognition, neurophysiology, and neurochemical pathways: A review." *Brain Plasticity (Amsterdam, Netherlands) 2*, 2, 127–152. doi: 10.3233/BPL-160040.
34　Giocomo, L.M. and Hasselmo, M.E. (2007) "Neuromodulation by glutamate and acetylcholine can change circuit dynamics by regulating the relative influence of afferent input and excitatory feedback." *Molecular Neurobiology 36*, 2, 184–200. doi: 10.1007/s12035-007-0032-z.
35　Conrad, C.D. (2008) "Chronic stress-induced hippocampal vulnerability: The glucocorticoid vulnerability hypothesis." *Reviews in the Neurosciences 19*, 6, 395–411. doi: 10.1515/revneuro.2008.19.6.395.
36　Tollenaar, M.S., Elzinga, B.M., Spinhoven, P., and Everaerd, W.A.M. (2008) "The effects of cortisol increase on long-term memory retrieval during and after acute psychosocial stress." *Acta Psychologica (Amsterdam) 127*, 3, 542–552. doi: 10.1016/j.actpsy.2007.10.007.
37　de Quervain, D.J., Roozendaal, B., Nitsch, R.M., McGaugh, J.L., and Hock, C. (2000) "Acute cortisone administration impairs retrieval of long-term declarative memory in humans." *Nature Neuroscience 3*, 4, 313–314. doi: 10.1038/73873.
38　Doidge, N. (2015) *The Brain's Way of Healing: Remarkable Discoveries and Recoveries from the Frontiers of Neuroplasticity*. London: Penguin Life, pp.11–20.
39　Fishman, L. and Ardman, C. (2012) *Yoga for Back Pain*. New York: W.W. Norton & Co., p.18.
40　Stanley, E. (2019) *Widen the Window: Training Your Brain and Body to Thrive During Stress and Recover from Trauma*. New York: Avery, pp.246, 253.
41　Brewer, J. (2021) *Unwinding Anxiety: New Science Shows How to Break the Cycles of Worry and Fear to Heal Your Mind*. New York: Avery, p.24.
42　van der Kolk, B. (2015) *The Body Keeps the Score: Brain, Mind and Body in the Healing of Trauma*. London: Penguin Publishing.
43　Rivest-Gadbois, E. and Boudrias, M.-H. (2019) "What are the known effects of yoga on the brain in relation to motor performances, body awareness and pain?" *Complementary Therapies in Medicine 44*, 129–142. doi: 10.1016/j.ctim.2019.03.021.
44　van der Kolk, B. (2015) *The Body Keeps the Score: Brain, Mind and Body in the Healing of Trauma*. London: Penguin Publishing, p.93.
45　Ogden, P. and Fisher, J. (2015) *Sensorimotor Psychotherapy: Interventions for Trauma and Attachment*. New York: W.W. Norton & Co., p.25.
46　van der Kolk, B. (2015) *The Body Keeps the Score: Brain, Mind and Body in the Healing of Trauma*. London: Penguin Publishing, p.207.
47　Buczynski, R., with van der Kolk, B. (2017) *How to Help Patients Rewire a Traumatized Brain*. Storrs, CT: NICABM (National Institute for the Clinical Application of Behavioral Medicine), p.7.
48　Buczynski, R., with van der Kolk, B. (2017) *How to Help Patients Rewire a Traumatized Brain*. Storrs, CT: NICABM (National Institute for the Clinical Application of Behavioral Medicine), p.7.

ENDNOTES

49 Desikachar, T.K.V. (1999) *The Heart of Yoga: Developing a Personal Practice*. Rochester, VT: Inner Traditions, p.51.
50 Porges, S. (2017) *Polyvagal Theory: Neurophysiological Foundations of Emotions, Attachment, Communication and Self-Regulation*. New York: W.W. Norton & Co, p.254.
51 Harvard Medical School (2016) *An Introduction to Yoga: Improve Your Strength, Balance, Flexibility, and Well-Being*. Boston, MA: Harvard Medical School Special Health Report, p.9.
52 Williams, K., Abildso, C., Steinberg, L., Doyle, E., Epstein, B., Smith, D., Hobbs, G., Gross, R., Kelley, G., and Cooper, L. (2009) "Evaluation of the effectiveness and efficacy of Iyengar Yoga." *Spine* 34, 19, 2066–2076. doi: 10.1097/BRS.0b013e3181b315cc
53 Villemure, C., Ceko, M., Cotton, V.A., and Bushnell, M.C. (2014) "Insular cortex mediates increased pain tolerance in yoga practitioners." *Cerebral Cortex* 24, 10, 2732–2740. doi: 10.1093/cercor/bht124.
54 US Department of Health and Human Services (2019) *Pain Management Best Practices Inter-Agency Task Force Report: Updates, Gaps, Inconsistencies, and Recommendations. Final Report*. May. www.hhs.gov/sites/default/files/pmtf-final-report-2019-05-23.pdf. p.43.
55 Chang, D.G., Holt, J.A., Sklar, M., and Groessl, E.J. (2016) "Yoga as a treatment for chronic low back pain: A systematic review of the literature." *Journal of Orthopedics and Rheumatology* 3, 1–8.
56 Cramer, H., Lauche, R., Haller, H., and Dobos, G. (2013) "A systematic review and meta-analysis of yoga for low back pain." *The Clinical Journal of Pain* 29, 5, 450–460. doi: 10.1097/AJP.0b013e31825e1492.
57 Groessl, E.J., Liu, L., Chang, D.G., Wetherell, J.L., et al. (2017) "Yoga for military veterans with chronic low back pain: A randomized clinical trial." *American Journal of Preventive Medicine* 53, 5, 599–608. doi: 10.1016/j.amepre.2017.05.019.
58 Saper, R.B., Lemaster, C., Delitto, A., Sherman, K.J., et al. (2017) "Yoga, physical therapy, or education for chronic low back pain: A randomized noninferiority trial." *Annals of Internal Medicine* 167, 2, 85–94. doi: 10.7326/M16-2579.
59 Cramer, H., Klose, P., Brinkhaus, B., Michalsen, A., and Dobos, G. (2017) "Effects of yoga on chronic neck pain: A systematic review and meta-analysis." *Clinical Rehabilitation* 31, 11, 1457–1465. doi: 10.1177/0269215517698735.
60 Wieland, L.S., Skoetz, N., Pilkington, S., Vempati, R., D'Adamo, C.R., and Berman, B.M. (2017) "Yoga treatment for chronic nonspecific low back pain." *Cochrane Database of Systematic Reviews* 1, 1, CD010671. doi: 10.1002/14651858.CD010671.pub2.
61 Cramer, H., Lange, S., Klose, P., Paul, A., and Dobos, G. (2012) "Yoga for breast cancer patients and survivors: A systematic review and meta-analysis." *BMC Cancer* 12, 412. doi: 10.1186/1471-2407-12-412.
62 Cramer, H., Lange, S., Klose, P., Paul, A., and Dobos, G. (2012) "Yoga for breast cancer patients and survivors: A systematic review and meta-analysis." *BMC Cancer* 12, 412. doi: 10.1186/1471-2407-12-412.
63 Merzenich, M. (2013) *Soft-Wired: How the New Science of Brain Plasticity Can Change Your Life*. San Francisco, CA: Parnassus Publishing, pp.232–241, p.233.
64 Merzenich, M. (2013) *Soft-Wired: How the New Science of Brain Plasticity Can Change Your Life*. San Francisco, CA: Parnassus Publishing, pp.232–241, p.233.
65 Merzenich, M. (2013) *Soft-Wired: How the New Science of Brain Plasticity Can Change Your Life*. San Francisco, CA: Parnassus Publishing, pp.232–241, p.241.
66 Merzenich, M. (2013) *Soft-Wired: How the New Science of Brain Plasticity Can Change Your Life*. San Francisco, CA: Parnassus Publishing, pp.232–241.

Chapter 4

1 Stanley, E. (2019) *Widen the Window: Training Your Brain and Body to Thrive During Stress and Recover from Trauma*. New York: Avery, p.315.
2 Lieberman, M.D. (2013) *Social: Why Our Brains Are Wired to Connect*. New York: Crown Books, Chapter 3.
3 Ogden, P. (2006) *Trauma and the Body: A Sensorimotor Approach to Psychotherapy*. New York: W.W. Norton & Co, p.146.
4 Levine, P. (2008) *Healing Trauma: A Pioneering Program for Restoring the Wisdom of Your Body*. Louisville, CO: Sounds True, p.30.

~ 271 ~

Chapter 5

1. Bell, C. (2007) *Mindful Yoga, Mindful Life: A Guide for Everyday Practice*. Boulder, CO: Shambhala Press, p.28.
2.
3.
4.
5. Porges, S. (2021) *Polyvagal Safety: Attachment, Communication, Self-Regulation*. New York: W.W. Norton & Co, p.263.
6. Herman, J. (1997) *Trauma and Recovery: The Aftermath of Violence—From Domestic Abuse to Political Terror*. New York: Basic Books, p.160.
7. Herman, J. (1997) *Trauma and Recovery: The Aftermath of Violence—From Domestic Abuse to Political Terror*. New York: Basic Books, p.133.
8. Emerson, D. and Hopper, E. (2011) *Overcoming Trauma Through Yoga*. Berkeley, CA: North Atlantic Books, pp.120–121.
9. Ogden, P. and Fisher, J. (2015) *Sensorimotor Psychotherapy: Interventions for Trauma and Attachment*. New York: W.W. Norton & Co, p.13.
10. Stanley, E. (2019) *Widen the Window: Training Your Brain and Body to Thrive During Stress and Recover from Trauma*. New York: Avery, p.246.
11. Emerson, D. and Hopper, E. (2011) *Overcoming Trauma Through Yoga*. Berkeley, CA: North Atlantic Books, p.56.
12. van der Kolk, B. (2015) *The Body Keeps the Score: Brain, Mind and Body in the Healing of Trauma*. London: Penguin Publishing, p.205.
13. van der Kolk, B. (2015) *The Body Keeps the Score: Brain, Mind and Body in the Healing of Trauma*. London: Penguin Publishing, p.205.
14. Erickson, M. (1982/1991) *My Voice Will Go With You: The Teaching Tales of Milton H. Erickson*. New York: W.W. Norton & Co.
15. Porges, S. (2017) *The Pocket Guide to Polyvagal Theory: The Transformative Power of Feeling Safe*. New York: W.W. Norton & Co., Chapters 1 and 5.
16. Porges, S. (2017) *The Pocket Guide to Polyvagal Theory: The Transformative Power of Feeling Safe*. New York: W.W. Norton & Co., pp.193–194.
17. Porges, S. (2017) *The Pocket Guide to Polyvagal Theory: The Transformative Power of Feeling Safe*. New York: W.W. Norton & Co., pp.47, 109, 141.
18. van der Kolk, B. (2015) *The Body Keeps the Score: Brain, Mind and Body in the Healing of Trauma*. London: Penguin Publishing, p.207.
19. Quoted in Keltner, D. (2009) *Born to Be Good: The Science of a Meaningful Life*. New York: W.W. Norton & Co, pp.28–29.
20. van der Kolk, B. (2015) *The Body Keeps the Score: Brain, Mind and Body in the Healing of Trauma*. London: Penguin Publishing, p.205.
21. Siegel, D. (2012/2020/2022) *The Developing Mind: How Relationships and the Brain Interact to Shape Who We Are*. New York: Guilford Press, pp.281–286.
22. Desikachar, T.K.V. (1999) *The Heart of Yoga: Developing a Personal Practice*. Rochester, VT: Inner Traditions, p.17.
23. Levine, P. (2008) *Healing Trauma: A Pioneering Program for Restoring the Wisdom of Your Body*. Louisville, CO: Sounds True, p.31.